THE VITAMIN CURE

for Children's Health Problems

RALPH K. CAMPBELL, M.D.,
AND ANDREW W. SAUL, PH.D.

Basic Health
PUBLICATIONS, INC.

The information contained in this book is based upon the research and personal and professional experiences of the authors. It is not intended as a substitute for consulting with your physician or other healthcare provider. Any attempt to diagnose and treat an illness should be done under the direction of a healthcare professional.

The publisher does not advocate the use of any particular healthcare protocol but believes the information in this book should be available to the public. The publisher and authors are not responsible for any adverse effects or consequences resulting from the use of the suggestions, preparations, or procedures discussed in this book. Should the reader have any questions concerning the appropriateness of any procedures or preparation mentioned, the authors and the publisher strongly suggest consulting a professional healthcare advisor.

Basic Health Publications, Inc.
www.basichealthpub.com

Library of Congress Cataloging-in-Publication Data

Campbell, Ralph K.
    The vitamin cure for children's health problems / Ralph K. Campbell and Andrew W. Saul. — 1st ed.
        p. cm.
    Includes bibliographical references and index.
    ISBN 978-1-59120-294-3 (Pbk.)
    ISBN 978-1-68162-825-7 (Hardcover)

    1. Orthomolecular therapy. 2. Children—Diseases—Alternative treatment. 3. Vitamin therapy. I. Saul, Andrew W. II. Title.

    RJ53.V57C36   2011
    615.3'28083—dc23

                                                    2011027745

Editor: John Anderson
Copyeditor: Peggy Hahn
Typesetting/Book design: Gary A. Rosenberg
Cover design: Mike Stromberg

CONTENTS

To Kenneth R. Campbell, our son, who was the "poster boy" for anti-ADHD believers. He embodied all the dynamic, positive traits of those given that label. And to my loving, supporting family, especially my extraordinarily patient wife, Jan.

—RALPH K. CAMPBELL

To my children, who took over my education long after I was done with college. And to Mrs. Edith Brewer, my first Sunday School teacher, who won me over by playing "Jingle Bells" on the piano for me every week, summer or winter.

—ANDREW W. SAUL

ACKNOWLEDGMENTS

We would like to thank the writers and editorial board of the Ortho-molecular Medicine News Service for their informative news releases, a number of which have been included in this book. We thank the International Schizophrenia Foundation and its Executive Director, Steven Carter, for kind permission to use material that was published in the *Journal of Orthomolecular Medicine*. We greatly appreciate the contributions to this book by Ian Brighthope, M.D., Robert G. Smith, Ph.D., William B. Grant, Ph.D., Steve Hickey, Ph.D., Hilary Roberts, Ph.D., and Damien Downing, M.D. Andrew Saul would especially like to thank his much better half, Colleen, for her unwavering support and loving encouragement. Ralph Campbell is indebted to his wife, Jan, for her support as a helpmate and a gourmet health-food cook.

FOREWORD

Allergies affect one in three children, asthma affects one in four children, attention-deficit hyperactivity disorder (ADHD) one in ten children, and autism nearly one in a hundred. Childhood cancers, obesity, diabetes, and depression have all more than doubled in the last two decades.

It is now said by many experts that the current generation of children may die before their parents or at an earlier age than the parents. It could also be said that despite the massive technological advances in medicine and health, the health and fitness of children in developed countries has been deteriorating at an increasing rate over the last few generations. The compelling evidence is clearly visible: we have a childhood obesity epidemic. Perhaps it's time to rethink our approach to medicine and health and revert to simpler, more commonsense approaches that have an evidence base but without the risks attached to modern medicine—for example, a megadose of vitamin A or D in the advent of a measles or influenza pandemic, respectively. The science is there to support such treatments.

The adults of today were adolescents and children not so long ago. If we had been more effective in getting across the message about nutritional (orthomolecular) medicine to the medical profession, the public, the government, and the media, we probably wouldn't be in the health mess we are today. We now have 26 million adults in America who have diabetes and 79 million more with pre-diabetes, conditions that raise the risk of developing heart disease and stroke.

These trends will continue if we cannot change attitudes and behaviors now.

Why write another book on vitamins or another book on children's health? Because no one has written a book about both so meaningfully, and in such a thoroughly readable form, regarding optimizing the health of children and the natural treatment of their common diseases. The authors have succeeded in making a potentially very heavy tome into a fascinating, realistic, and scientifically factual read.

THINK FOR YOURSELF

I cannot tell you how many children I have seen who have attended one of the best children's hospitals in the world, suffering from severe eczema, sterile abscesses, or pathological constipation, and who had been fed fortified cow's milk in the hospital. On discharge after surgery and on massive doses of cortisone, these children remain on cow's milk, only to be readmitted with the same problems. A simple elimination of cow's milk and the eczema clears, the sterile abscesses heal, and no more constipation. There are other benefits also, including improvements in learning, behavior, and immunity.

Unfortunately, modern medicine no longer deserves the trust of many patients, as it has become fundamentally based on misinformation, arrogance, and ignorance fostered by a system geared to pharmaceutical interests. It is even worse when it comes to the health care of our children and the prescription of toxic drugs for the treatment of viral infections with antibiotics, ADHD with stimulants, and mood disorders with antidepressants.

One of the pioneers in vitamin therapy, Linus Pauling, wrote that the human body and mind could be made disease free and heal themselves if the correct concentration of all nutrients were provided. It makes a lot of sense. Dr. Pauling's philosophy can be summed up as, "Never put your trust in anything but your own intellect—always think for yourself." I believe that this book offers to all parents the facts upon which they can base trust in their own intellect to achieve optimum health care and the best outcomes for their children. When it comes to the care of your children, think for yourself.

A RIGHT TO EFFECTIVE CARE

Patients have a right to the safest, cheapest, and most ethical effective care. This is an essential right for all people, including children, neonates, and the unborn. Patients and their parents or guardians have clear rights to refuse medical treatments, but there are no express rights to demand a course of treatment of a particular kind—this is a major weakness in virtually every health-care system in the developed world. Health practitioners have no express obligation to comply with a patient's demand for a particular course of treatment. Patients generally have rights to give or withhold informed consent and be provided with information about potential treatments. Ideally, this should include effective, safe alternative and complementary modalities.

Additionally, we need an attitudinal change in the medical establishment, particularly in the medical schools, and a retraining of the medical profession. A focus on nutrition and lifestyle issues at medical school and a requirement that continuing education points be achieved through learning about prevention of chronic diseases is imperative, and if the medical profession is too reluctant to embrace these developments, others will fill the gaps. Sadly, most continuing education that doctors receive is about new drugs, and this has contributed to reducing the doctor's role to that of prescription writer.

Health care is more than that: optimum health should be the objective for everyone. Once a person is diagnosed with a disease, the costs begin to add up. While the monetary cost is certainly substantial, the human toll of pain and suffering, and the impact on productivity and the lives of friends and relatives, can be shattering. Health is difficult to sell, as it is human nature to take something for granted if it is functioning. In many cases, the killer diseases—heart disease, cancer, stroke, diabetes, asthma, and depression—are the culmination of many years of easy effort. This book goes a long way to show that it is easier, in the long run, to stay healthy.

There is a paucity of scientific medical evidence to support the majority of present-day medical practices, many of which could be replaced by safer, more economical, and more sensible nutritional and orthomolecular medicine practices. These practices are brilliantly covered in this book by two very experienced clinicians and authors. The future of human health is a gamble and the odds are stacked against us. Drs. Campbell and Saul have delivered a real solution to reduce those odds.

—Ian Brighthope, M.D.

INTRODUCTION

It is a curious fact that both of the authors have worked in prisons (and no, not as inmates). Dr. Campbell was a prison physician and I (AWS) was a prison college instructor. Dr. Campbell, in my opinion, is much like well-known children's doctor Lendon H. Smith in that both of them came to nutritional (orthomolecular) practice later in their professional lives. The thirty-five years I have in natural health education, and Dr. Campbell's forty-plus years of experience as a board-certified pediatrician, motivate us to share a useful message with you—nutrition prevents and cures illness.

You have already noticed that this book is neither thick nor technical. This is not a textbook and it is not meant to be a comprehensive overview of all children's health problems. It is, however, a practical guide to using therapeutic nutrition (orthomolecular medicine) specifically where it works best. There are a number of common childhood illnesses that can be prevented and effectively treated with vitamins and other nutrients. We focus on these in this text. As you use nutrition more and more, you may experience, as I did as a young father, that there are side benefits instead of side effects. I repeatedly saw so many health issues fade to the vanishing point that my children literally never met their pediatrician. Of course, they had annual physicals at school, and we had the physician's phone number on our fridge if we needed it. The secret is not about refusing to go to a pediatrician—the secret is to not need to go.

The details of this secret are not automatically manifested. Rather, it requires time investment and ongoing learning. Many years ago, my mother (who had been a teacher) told me that *education should make you want to learn more.* When I was a kid, I had too much time on my hands in the summer and was bored out of my mind in school all winter. I did not appreciate this then, but we all have the same twenty-four hours in each day. Most of us (and even the busiest of people) have time for TV or certain other pursuits. Taking a bit of that time to learn to get well and stay well is the most certain of all investments. Consider this: if you are pressed for time, but spend some fraction of an hour each day improving your health, you will probably live longer. If you live longer, then you will have more time in the end. Now, decades later, I see what Mom was on to.

WHAT'S AHEAD

This book is divided into four parts.

- Part One: Nutrition or Medicines? introduces the concept of therapeutic nutrition and taking control of your family's health. It covers the issues of antibiotics and vaccinations and looks at natural ways to boost immune function.

- Part Two: Staying Healthy with Diet and Detoxification provides information on healthy eating for children and covers the topic of cholesterol and children. It also takes and in-depth look at the dangers of toxins in the environment.

- Part Three: Major Children's Health Problems tackles three of the most pressing health issues for children: obesity and diabetes, allergies and asthma, and attention-deficit hyperactivity disorder (ADHD).

- Part Four: Vitamin Therapy provides guidance on using therapeutic doses of vitamin C and other nutrients.

The additional reading suggested at the end of this book is especially important, for in seeking you will gain much more really helpful information than this book can hold. When I was in college, often as bored as before, some instructors said—and a few actually meant—that *education should teach you to think for yourself.* When we just "go to the doctor," we are suspending most thought and asking to be commanded. Like a toddler putting up his arms to have you take off his shirt, we surrender our self-reliance for some quick service. We also get to complain if the treatment wasn't good enough for us.

I once heard a person complaining that firefighters had tracked mud and water into her living room en route downstairs to a small smolder in the basement clothes dryer. A firefighter responded, "Look, lady, when you call the fire department, your house is ours." Similarly, when you call the doctor, you give up control of your very body. To keep control as parents, we have to become more educated and more self-reliant. This book is, we hope, a helpful step in that direction.

PART ONE

NUTRITION
OR DRUGS?

CHAPTER 1

DISCOVERING THE POWER OF VITAMINS AND OTHER NUTRIENTS

"No illness which can be treated by diet
should be treated by any other means."
—MOSES MAIMONIDES (1135–1204)

What a tough job it is being a good parent. A conscientious parent loses confidence from all the authoritative push of "experts" to treat everything with drugs, while putting little emphasis on unhealthy diets and minimizing the value of vitamin supplements. Are parents to believe the "science" or go by instinctive common sense, perhaps engendered by their own parents?

I (RC) was a practicing pediatrician for over forty years. The "good old days" might just be a once-in-a-lifetime experience, but that doesn't mean they should pass away unappreciated. With careful examination of the past, we might find some real treasures. Once I hung up my stethoscope, I ceased to be a voice of authority except for a few parents or grandparents of my former pediatric patients, whom I see in the grocery store. The good side of this is that I have time to tie together my experiences in examining environmental toxins, nutrition, and medical care—to synthesize what was working in a rewarding practice with what I feel is lacking in practice today. Studying the science behind nutritional biochemistry is the only way to evaluate the worth, or lack of it, of a nutrient or a drug.

People who are aware of only the last twenty years of medical and nutritional science are seeing just a small part of the picture. I know

6

there is no way to completely return to the "good old days," nor should we. We shouldn't disregard the rescue value of some surgeries or some medicines any more than we should completely disregard what we have learned in the past concerning how to achieve and maintain health. I have come to appreciate the maxim of orthomolecular medicine pioneer Abram Hoffer, M.D.: when speaking of alternative medicine, nutrition should be the primary, and medicine the alternative.

> *Orthomolecular* means the "right molecule" or "correct molecule." Conventional pharmaceuticals, such as chemotherapy, tend to be "toximolecular." Vitamins and insulin are examples of orthomolecular therapeutic substances. Throughout this book, we will refer to the principle of orthomolecular medicine: using an *optimal* dose of the *right* molecule.

FINDING REAL TREASURES

When I was a child, I never considered it "uncool" to have an eagerness to learn, especially of anything resembling science. I grew up in a period that coincided with the heyday of vitamin research, the 1930s and 1940s. Both yesterday and today, children often need a kick to send them off in the right direction. My "kickoff" was provided by my mother, who gave me a two-volume book called *Man in Structure and Function* (New York: Knopf, 1943). A large part of the first volume was devoted to vitamins. I was thrilled. *Vita*-min sounds a lot like *vital*. I got the picture: vitamins are vital if we want to live. We have to get them from our diet since our bodies cannot manufacture them.

Believe it or not, for me, *Man in Structure and Function* was more exciting than books on any other subject, even dinosaurs. I learned about the deficiency diseases: beriberi, rickets, and scurvy. I discovered that, in the 1600s, sailors on long voyages suffered from the ravages of scurvy—bleeding into soft tissues, including gums (with teeth falling out), painful joints, internal bleeding. Gross, but fascinating. It turned out that scurvy was due to lack of a substance (now known to be vitamin C) in the diet; after their bodily stores of the vitamin were gone (in about six weeks), sailors began to experience scurvy symptoms. Scottish physician James Lind (1716–1794) eventually showed that citrus fruit could cure scurvy. The first fix involved fruits and vitamin C–containing vegetables such as cabbage and "scurvy grass" sorrel. Prevention was later focused on citrus fruits. Hence, the common moniker for the British sailor at the time, "limey."

Massive changes take place in one's life from the first year of high school to the final year of medical school. During this busy time, I crammed my mind so full of facts in preparation for and completion of medical school that, to avoid overflow, I paid no attention to increasing my nutrition knowledge. The frantic search for "practical" knowledge, necessary for practicing medicine, prevailed in medical schools of the day. Like most new doctors, I had gained very little new knowledge of nutrition and health factors from instruction in medical school. Internship and residency training spun the wheels even faster—with so many facts pouring in, and so much work to do, there was little time for reflection.

AN AWAKENING OF THINKING

Change for the better came when I began to apply what I had learned in the actual practice of pediatrics. Starting with my first week of practice, I gained a wealth of knowledge from a devoted newborn nursery nurse, and the dormant nutrition segment of my brain was aroused again. She had all the doctors who placed newborns in her care firmly under her wing, and we prescribed a vitamin drop for each baby, containing vitamins A, D, and C. Concomitant with what I gained from people "in the trenches" was what I read in my specialty journal, *Pediatrics*. At that time, a pediatric practice was predicated on the so-called "well-baby checkup," so there were many articles that provided sound nutritional advice, including some from greats like Nobel Prize winner Albert Szent-Györgyi, who isolated and synthesized vitamin C.

These factors—readily available, honest literature and real-world, hands-on experience—got the snowball rolling and growing. For a while, there was a balance in the literature and in pediatric seminars between nutrition's part in healthy living and medicine's part. Then, in the 1950s and 1960s, there began to be a profound shift of emphasis: more and more on medicines, less and less on nutrition.

Ironically, at about the same time, there was an awakening of thinking about foods and everything else we put into our bodies, and it became clear that what we eat has a lot to do with our health. The first myth to come under the gun was everybody's staple, "enriched" white flour. This "enriched" myth was long-standing and had achieved a sort of squatter's rights that could hardly be challenged. I've often wondered, if all things were equal in terms of endured hardships, who would have been more healthy in the last half of the nineteenth century in France and Britain—the country peasants or the city-dwellers? The bread containing "refined" wheat flour was more in vogue in the city than with the dwellers of the countryside, whose sustaining peasant bread was more like the real thing. Indeed, one account has it that the original white bread was a cosmetic novelty, a royalist party favor to show support for the French king. White was the traditional color of the French monarch, so palace guests wore white clothes, sported white powdered hair, and ate white bread.

Of course, milled and bleached flour cannot support life. So, later, thanks to the work of Joseph Goldberger, M.D., white flour was enriched with some of what had been taken from it when it was first "de-riched." When the bran, with its fiber and trace mineral content and the germ (the source of vitamin E and several B vitamins) are removed in milling, only the starchy, denuded endosperm remains. Why this dastardly deed? The sole reason is to increase product shelf life. In the days of the Industrial Revolution, too much time elapsed from production to the marketplace to prevent oxidation of the fatty components of whole wheat. The result was an unmarketable, rancid product. Also, when the nutrients were removed, ants and weevils had nothing to do with this "non-food" food. Smart critters!

ORTHOMOLECULAR MEDICINE PIONEER: JOSEPH GOLDBERGER, M.D.

It is still true today what Hugh Riordan, M.D., said some years back: "Orthomolecular is not the answer to any question posed in medical school." Such was most definitely the case in 1895, when Joseph Goldberger (1874–1929) completed his medical degree, with honors, at Bellevue Hospital Medical School in New York. After private practice and a stint working as a quarantine officer on Ellis Island, Dr. Goldberger became an expert in infectious diseases. At the time, pellagra was believed to be infectious, and people suffering from the condition were treated as if they were lepers. Attempts were made to deny their children admittance to public school. The disease was thought to be so contagious that it was not uncommon for people with pellagra to be refused hospital admission.

The justification was official: in 1914, a governmental commission declared that pellagra appeared to be infectious and that it certainly had nothing to do with diet. That same year, the U.S. Public Health service assigned Dr. Goldberger to the problem, and things began to look up. Dr. Goldberger had the very politically incorrect idea that pellagra was related to the malnutrition of poverty. He personally observed what patients ate, and concluded that the cause of this tragedy was the "three M's": a tryptophan- and niacin-deficient diet of some fatty *meat*, some *molasses*, and a whole lot of corn *meal*.

Today, it is sometimes forgotten just how big the tragedy actually was. In addition to the infamous "three D" symptoms of pellagra (*d*iarrhea, *d*ermatitis, and *d*ementia), there is a fourth "D": death. It was as difficult then as it is now to think that a nutrient deficiency could kill. Well, it can, and it did. Of 3 million American cases of pellagra in the first half of the twentieth century, some 100,000 people died from it.[1] A far higher number were disabled by mental illness.

In later years, we learned that the solution is supplementation with a vitamin: nicotinic acid or niacin. Simple? Fictional sleuth Sherlock Holmes was given to saying that "all problems are simple when they are explained." But in 1914, the year World War One began, science was winging it. I (AWS) used to tell my students that science is built upon the mistakes of those who came before us. Not this time. Dr. Goldberger was innovative and orthomolecular, and he got it right the first time. Goldberger believed that the amino acid tryptophan was likely the "pellagra-preventive factor" and that upplemental yeast was the therapy. He was right on both counts. In weeks, he cured pellagra in children, prisoners, and psychotics.

As Dr. Hoffer said: "In the early 1940s, the United States government mandated the addition of niacinamide to flour. This eradicated the terrible pandemic of pellagra in just two years, and ought to be recognized as the most successful public health measure for the elimination of a major disease in psychiatry, the pellagra psychoses. The reaction of contemporary physicians was predictable. Indeed, at the time, Canada rejected the idea and declared the addition of vitamins to flour to be an adulteration."[2]

Dr. Hoffer, a cereal biochemistry Ph.D. as well as a loyal Canadian, saw it first-hand. Today, Health Canada glosses over the embarrassing fact that, in 1942, the government had said: "The use of synthetic vitamins in the manufacture of flour or bread for sale for consumption in Canada is hereby expressly declared to be an adulteration of food." Indeed, throughout the 1930s, Canadian nutrition authorities were skeptical of adding vitamins to the average diet, in spite of the fact that enrichment of flour began in the U.S. as early as 1938.[3] It was not until 1976 that enrichment of flour at the mill level with thiamine, riboflavin, niacin, and iron became mandatory nationwide in Canada. The latest addition to white flour is folic acid, designed to prevent spina bifida, a deformity of the newborn. Dr. Hoffer would probably agree that consumption of "whole" foods would have prevented these deficiency diseases. Adding these essential nutrients to depleted foods is a necessary stopgap measure until better eating habits in the general population can be developed.

Knowledge comes at a cost: Dr. Goldberger had yellow fever, dengue, and very nearly died of typhus. The U.S. National Institutes of Health says he "stepped on Southern pride when he linked the poverty of Southern sharecroppers, tenant farmers, and mill workers to the deficient diet that caused pellagra."[4] In the end, Dr. Goldberger was nominated for the Nobel Prize. Had he not died earlier in the year, he might well have shared it in 1929 with vitamin researchers Christiaan Eijkman and Frederick G. Hopkins.

Dr. Goldberger was a great public health pioneer who went against conventional medicine when he insisted, unto his death, that a dreadful, fatal disease could be treated simply "by varying the concentration in the human body of substances that are normally present in the body." That is Linus Pauling's own definition of orthomolecular medicine. Of course, Pauling had just turned 13 when Goldberger first practiced it.

After some vitamins were isolated and could be synthesized (in the 1930s and 1940s), a few of the cheaper B vitamins were added back to refined flour, as was iron—thus, we had so-called enriched flour. But prior to this slight enlightenment, the perpetrators had no idea that they were throwing the nutrients away by refining the flour. Commercial gain from augmenting shelf life was the reasonable thing to do; whole-grain flour would not keep. The final insult to refined flour came in the form of bleaching with various organic peroxides or chlorine, providing a more "pure" appearance, since the refining process itself left a "yellowish" appearance to the product.

I have devoted some space to this problem, since it perhaps represents the first classic instance of nutrition "science," or what Michael Pollan, in his book *In Defense of Food*, calls "nutritionism."[5] According to Pollan, food science practitioners think they can improve upon nature by extracting nutrients from a food and recombining them into a superior product—"superior" in appearance and in reducing spoilage (and salability). Great effort was made not only to sell the product, but to sell the *idea* of nutrition science. Back when "Wonder Bread," the super-refined white bread wrapped in a package studded with colorful balloons, claimed that their bread "builds bodies 12 ways," some of us could think of only four: wide, thick, flabby, and weak. For years, nutrition advocate Carlton Fredericks, Ph.D., staunchly opposed and lampooned it, and refined white bread in general, on coast-to-coast radio. Critics of the food industry were labeled "food faddists," a marginalizing term that persists to this day.

Since the "bread of life," a prime staple in the diets of many cultures, was now itself on life support, the resuscitation process was initiated. Small, independent bakeries began producing whole-grain breads, with which one could put together a sandwich full of newly rediscovered "whole" foods. Many switched from white to more "natural" bread, mainly because they felt this would be a move that would better their health, but what a pleasant surprise to find that the new bread tasted great, too. For many "meat and potato" types, the priorities were switched: it tastes great and the extra perk is that it is also healthier.

If it is tough for adults to make the transition, we assume it will be tougher for children. The solution lies in the presentation by a parent who wants the best for his or her children and wants them to willingly accept new things that are good for them. With this proper atmosphere, it is amazing how easily "yuk" turns to "yum." The children are nutritionally launched into a lifetime of healthier eating.

I am fortunate to have a wife with an innate sense of what constitutes good food, who is at the same time an imaginative gourmet cook. Much like in the parent-child scenario described above, she converted me during this whole food renaissance of the 1960s, and I soon embraced the many benefits of the movement, including redoubling my interest in vitamins.

VITAMIN SUPPLEMENTATION IN ACTION

Then came the exciting change of location and life—my move to the great state of Montana in 1970. Initially, I conducted well-child checkups for Native Americans and pediatric consultations for the local medical doctors. Very soon, it was apparent that these services should be part of a county health department service for all. Volunteers went door to door, canvassing every seventh registered voter to determine if there was support for this idea. As a result of this polling, a county nurse was hired and a department was formed. This was the start of my "adult medicine" education, which opened my eyes to the imperative need for nutrition education in this expanded population. My study was spurred on by the questions from those I treated or, more often, those I just listened to.

When I became the doctor for the local detention center (jail), I really had an eye-opener. If the inmate had a doctor out in the real world, I was to honor that doctor by trying to continue their care plan as much as possible. The thing that shocked me was discovering how many inmates were on dangerous prescribed medications and didn't even know it. They often didn't know the names of the drugs

ORTHOMOLECULAR MEDICINE PIONEER: CARLTON FREDERICKS, PH.D.

Carlton Fredericks (1910–1987), born Harold Carlton Caplan, grew up in Brooklyn, New York, and received a master's degree in 1949 and a doctorate in 1955, in Public Health Education from New York University. He wrote over twenty books, lectured widely, and was Associate Professor of Public Health at Fairleigh Dickinson University in New Jersey.

Dr. Fredericks became famous—and in some circles, infamous—for his pioneering use of the media to educate people about vitamin and nutrition therapy. On the radio for nearly half a century, his nationally syndicated call-in "Design for Living" program resulted in millions of letters to a man whom many considered "America's Foremost Nutritionist." KABC Los Angeles presented his program "Living Should Be Fun" saying that, "Dr. Fredericks presents interviews with doctors and nutritionists (and) examines the fact or superstition in certain nutrition beliefs."

Dr. Fredericks, a colleague of Drs. Robert Atkins and Linus Pauling, was heavily criticized as a vitamin "promoter" and food "faddist." He constantly made fun of junk foods and brought his listeners many a memorable moment. He quipped that if you lack they were taking, and usually hadn't a clue of what the drug was for. Worse still, very few had any notion of what constituted a good diet, particularly the need for optimal vitamin intake. Most were incarcerated for alcohol- and/or drug-related problems. In time, depending on the duration of the inmate's problems, I could predict the nutritional deficiencies by inspection of body build, coloring, the condition of teeth and gums, attitude, and other physical and psychological characteristics. I don't have a formula for aging, but most of the prisoners were definitely "old" for their chronological age.

I instituted a program for all incoming inmates: a multivitamin-mineral tablet and chewable tablet of vitamin C (500 mg) daily as

the time to learn what you ought to know about healthy eating, just follow the average grocery store shopper and purchase only what he or she doesn't. When callers asked about white bread, he replied that it "makes a wonderful way of cleaning off your countertops. You can dust your furniture with it."

In the early 1970s, one of the first nutrition zingers I (AWS) ever read was Dr. Fredericks' comment in *Food Facts and Fallacies* that diabetics could be weaned off of insulin with extremely high doses of B-complex vitamins. One may reasonably entertain doubts if a type 1 diabetic could ever be free of the need to take insulin. On the other hand, I have seen diabetics require significantly less insulin when they take a high-potency B-complex supplement every two to three hours. The action is so profound that diabetics need to demand a suitably cautious therapeutic trial, with insulin dosage adjustment made and supervised by their physician.

Searching the shelves back in 1945, you would have found that one of Dr. Fredericks's first books was entitled *Living Should Be Fun*. Forty years later, the title of one of his last books was *Arthritis: Don't Learn to Live with It*. The man was nothing if not consistent. He promoted life and health, asserting that you needed vitamin supplements for both.

standard treatment. The alcoholics were given a B-50 preparation (B-complex vitamins) daily, as well; many, especially those with gum disease, also took 400 IU of natural (d-tocopherol) vitamin E once a day. I would have liked to prescribe considerably more vitamin C, and I did administer 1,000 mg three times a day for any postsurgical patients to aid healing. I was amazed in witnessing a tooth socket, left vacant from an extraction, almost filling in as I watched, when I provided this much vitamin C and vitamin E.

There were clear benefits of vitamin supplementation that accrued to the inmate:

- He or she could more easily withdraw from alcohol or drugs. Plus, if they were in long enough, they just plain felt better, a big factor in attitude adjustment and a gain of energy.

- I worked with the cook in order to provide the best diet that would be allowed under a stingy budget. Healthy food was foreign to many of the inmates.

- If I could convince them of the benefits of exercise, the good feeling increased to the point of thinking about lifestyle changes.

I would encourage the inmates to continue the regimen when released. Without these steps, I knew we would likely see them behind bars again, malnourished and back to square one. I was so dismayed to find that, even after my explanation of why I prescribed these vitamins, many regarded these nutrients as just "more pills." Worse, the jailers felt the same way and restricted my "prescriptions." They were considered just another excess budget item. The department never hesitated paying for expensive—and often worthless—medications, but regarded a vitamin as a superfluous medication. That is how profound the ignorance was and how naive I had been.

DEEPENING NUTRITIONAL KNOWLEDGE

My frustration grew and "jailhouse lawyers" set their wrath upon me. This was one of the best things that could have happened, as it resulted in my resigning and spurred my zeal to help fill the nutritional knowledge vacuum. I got the attention of William Crook, M.D., when we were both published in the "Letters to the Editors" section of *Pediatrics*. We found that we were in agreement concerning the cause of the nebulous syndrome attention deficit disorder (ADD). Dr. Crook was a Fellow of the American Academy of Pediatrics (AAP) and a member of the American College of Allergists and the Society of Clinical Ecology.

Our correspondence led to an invitation to a meeting of clinical ecologists, of which Dr. Crook was a ranking member. Their thrust was threefold: nutrition, allergy, and toxicology.[6] Learning about their approach bolstered my concepts of allergy problems. The toxicology studies that were presented greatly aided my continuing public health endeavors—such topics as "toxic building syndrome" and lead and pesticide toxicity proved essential. Best of all, the nutrition presentations inspired me to learn more and to apply what I already had learned.

William Osler, M.D., famous for his clinic in New Orleans, once wrote that he was "well aware that the patient's bedside was the chief arena of medical education." Substitute "bedside" with "office setting" and that reinforced my thought of learning from my patients. By listening to mothers, concepts like "allergic tension-fatigue syndrome" made more sense; there is a strong food allergy–behavior tie.

I also became familiar with Jack Challem, who abstracted nutrition articles and published them in a monthly newsletter, *Nutrition Reporter*. He also gave talks at the Orthomolecular Medicine Today conferences and is author of several books. When Jack sent me a copy of his newsletter, I responded with an enthusiastic letter, stating that this was just what I was looking for. He allowed me to supply him with home-spun ideas I had gleaned and developed from past experience and the sparse literature of the time. I found that Jack Challem, Dr. Crook, and Dr. Lendon Smith, a pediatrician who had a popular television broadcast from Oregon, all had a common interest in promoting these ideas.

In the 1990s, I got a computer with Internet capabilities and, at about the same time, an invitation from Jack to attend an Orthomol-

ORTHOMOLECULAR MEDICINE PIONEER: LENDON SMITH, M.D.

Lendon Smith (1921–2001), the man who would become nationally known as "The Children's Doctor," received his M.D. in 1946 from the University of Oregon Medical School. In 1955, Dr. Smith became Clinical Professor of Pediatrics at the University of Oregon Hospital. He would practice pediatrics for thirty-five years before retiring in 1987 to lecture, write, and help make "megavitamin" a household word.

And yet it was not until after twenty years of medical practice that Dr. Smith first began to use megavitamin therapy. A patient "wanted me to give her a vitamin shot," he wrote of an alcoholic woman from 1973. "I had never done such a useless thing in my professional life, and I was a little embarrassed to think that she considered me to be the kind of doctor who would do that sort of thing."[7] As it turned out, "that sort of thing" consisted of an intramuscular injection of B-complex vitamins, which proved successful enough that "she walked past three bars and didn't have to go in." This was the beginning of his evolution from conventional pediatrician to orthomolecular spokesperson.

His first book, *The Children's Doctor* (1969), contains only three mentions of vitamins, and two are negative. But as Dr. Smith learned about megavitamin therapy, he began to discuss it. In *Feed Your Kids Right* (1979), he recommends up to 10,000 mg of vitamin C during illness. Just two years later, in *Foods for Healthy Kids* (1981), he now recommends vitamin C to bowel tolerance levels. But even his relatively mild statements, such as "eat no sugar" and "stress increases the need for vitamin B and C, calcium, magnesium, and zinc" can be a walk on the wild side for pharmaphilic physicians. And Smith's *Feed Yourself Right* recommendations for B-complex and vitamin C injections, self-administered by the patient twice a week for three weeks, are not calculated to dodge controversy.[8]

Dr. Smith couldn't have cared less about his critics, and by 1979, he was a *New York Times* best-selling author. By 1983, he was an advocate of four-day water fasts, 1,000 microgram injections of B_{12}, and megavitamins for kids. There were no RDA-level vitamin recommendations to be found in a Lendon Smith book. He was an outspoken critic of junk food—two of his trademark phrases were: "People tend to eat the food to which they are sensitive" and "If you love something, it is probably bad for you."

Dr. Smith was one of the first to unambiguously support high-dose vitamin regimens for children. Such a position did not endear him to fellow members of the American Academy of Pediatrics, and it is therefore further to his credit that he boldly stepped forward and took orthomolecular therapy directly to the people. In this he was particularly successful, achieving renown by way of his newsletter (*The Facts*) and his many popular books, articles, videos, and prime-time television appearances.[9]

ecular Medicine Today conference. There I was immersed in many ideas and concepts of nutritional health that I had previously dug out of almost nowhere. Everything was crystallized and presented in a way I could digest. This and subsequent meetings put me into a different realm of knowledge and curiosity. It was almost like a support group to help me discern the truths about achieving and maintaining health. I began to realize that, as a physician, I had not really paid attention to the way established medicine disparaged the well-documented truths of orthomolecular medicine, in order to defend its turf. Those quick to dismiss nutrition therapy tried to turn the tables, and put orthomolecular medicine practitioners on the defensive.

In this great "information age," we all have difficulty discerning the truth, especially when making money becomes a prime motive to express a viewpoint. Examining nutrition articles is particularly hard. Depending on the bias of the author of nutritional information—for or against—powerful arguments are made. But strength or volume of the viewpoint does not determine truth.

Here is how I treat a nutrition article from mainstream medicine: if I find the authors have experience and integrity, and that what they have proposed has had enough trials to show that it is safe, I will put it into my mental "useful" file. I open this "file" whenever I come upon similar material to see if the new material withstands scrutiny. I think this will work for anyone who has the necessary balance of open-mindedness and a necessary modicum of skepticism.

SUMMARY

Dr. Campbell discovered the power of therapeutic nutrition (orthomolecular medicine) by seeing the difference it can make in people's lives. You, too, can discover the healing potential found in safe, effective vitamins, minerals, and other natural supplements. As a parent, you want to provide the best care possible for your children. Therapeutic nutrition is something you can learn about and begin to use today.

CHAPTER 2

GO TO THE DOCTOR OR BECOME THE DOCTOR?

"The medical profession [is] a conspiracy to hide its own shortcomings. No doubt the same may be said of all professions. They are all conspiracies against the laity."
—GEORGE BERNARD SHAW (1856–1950)

NUTRITION OR DRUGS?

Can you picture this? A charge of $5 to $8 for a visit to the pediatrician for an acute problem, or $15 for a half-hour visit for a new patient or for an established patient with a more complex problem. The extra time is needed for gathering input from the parent, a comprehensive physical exam, and outlining a solution that included written directions that reinforced the conversation. A new mother could have a private room on the obstetrics wing of the hospital for $20 a day. Necessary tests were inexpensive and parents (pre–medical insurance times) could easily shoulder the cost.

Yes, it happened. Go back with time warp to the post–World War II days when families never had it so good. Disciplined young men who had been discharged from the military were eager to work, marry, and raise a family, and had every opportunity to get on with fulfilling those wishes or to first enter college (paid for under the GI Bill). The American dream of owning a house was soon realized for many. Our great economy supplied the thriving industrial world with automobiles, home appliances, construction equipment, and even some newly developed electronic "wonders" such as television, all of which created well-paying jobs for those who were willing to work. Income was relatively high and expenses were low, so it was easy to earn a "living wage." With the end of the war, mothers rarely considered working outside the home.

But things would change. Previously unchallenged, the common-sense approach toward achieving worthwhile goals of daily living soon gave way to embracing the "new," especially those things with a "science" spin to them. Processed foods, scientifically assembled, flooded the marketplace. Our appetite for comfort grew. Now, we *needed* a TV, a good car (or two), distant vacations, and a comfortable home. The solution was to create the two-salary household. The catch-22 was that an increase in household income was coupled with increased household costs (daycare, wardrobe, transportation). "Science" became synonymous with "modern," while the old ways too often were regarded as just that—old.

By definition, science is "a branch of knowledge or study dealing with a body of facts or truths systematically arranged and showing the operation of general laws." It is increasingly difficult today to capture a degree of discernment necessary to clearly define *facts, truths,* or *general laws,* due to our brains being flooded with information from television, the Internet, and other media. Even new knowledge under the umbrella of "science" requires discernment accompanied by a healthy dose of skeptical scrutiny. The recent mapping of the human genome was a wonderful thing and has great potential for providing clues for disease diagnosis and occasionally for treatment. But this has been sensationalized; what *might* be is not *now.*

What we have now, and have had for decades, is knowledge of how to enhance the workings of many genes through diet and supplements and the avoidance of toxic substances. Let us not be so enamored with science that we ignore what is working, if we will just let it. Just as the followers of food science had convinced the public that they could reassemble nutrients to form a food superior to one from nature, so have medical science's followers been successful in convincing the public that, through research, they can devise medicines to treat every disease or disorder in a way that would be superior to a nutritional approach.

Madison Avenue Medicine

This change in attitude accelerated greatly over the last twenty years, as pharmaceutical medicine became an ever more powerful industry rather than a service. Today, at least one out of every four children or teenagers is taking a medication to treat a chronic condition, most commonly depression, asthma, or attention deficit. The medical establishment has been very successful in progressively strengthening this image and putting nutrition therapy on the back burner. Following the Madison Avenue tactics of other industries, the medical industry proceeded full steam ahead with advertising for medicines, hospitals and clinics, and physicians, in every form of media. First of all, the time-honored taboo set by medical organizations, such as the American Medical Association, that condemned advertising for doctors, had to be put aside. The industry concept was further strengthened by the introduction of health care insurance, an industry in itself.

I experienced a perfect illustration of the effectiveness of the pharmaceutical industry's brainwashing campaign. While shopping at my local supermarket, I was carrying a bottle of vitamin E when I met a couple my age, who were the parents of one of my pediatric patients years before, coming down the aisle. Her comment was, "More pills?" I said, "Capsules of a very important substance much better than pills—vitamin E. Fortunately, I don't have to take any medications." She said, "Well, Bob had a heart attack so, of course, he has to take Plavix." Can we please turn back the clock?

Medical care is now just another advertised product to hawk. What does a typical medical television ad depict? Does it show a compassionate doctor sitting with a patient explaining the findings and treatment plan derived from the current visit and actually using the stethoscope? No! More likely it will show an operating room scene with gowned and masked individuals hovering over a patient surrounded by a multiplicity of tubes and machines.

How did the patient get there in the first place? Surgical techniques and diagnostic imaging procedures are as good or better in this country than anywhere else in the world, but access to these services is through a primary doctor or other medical professional. Also, this doctor is the one to write a prescription; the patient also needs the means to fill it. There is a need for a personal physician to pull together all specialty referrals and tests, much like a construction contractor in charge of sub-contracting. The "personal" primary doctor should be equipped to field questions like: "What is really happening to joints that, like car parts, they far too often have to be replaced?" "Why is there so much cancer?" "Why are so many hearts in need of surgical intervention?" "Are these things inevitable or can we work together to improve our odds?" And the big question: *"Why can't I try nutritional remedies first before being put on medicines fraught with dangerous side effects?"*

A good piece of the answer lies in the fact that a primary doctor, under the gun of the insurance carrier, is not being allowed sufficient time, either with patients or for study. The razzle-dazzle of the "science" behind medicines, accompanied by surgical and diagnostic imaging techniques, trumps seeing the necessity of more time spent with patients. Time spent is not just for building rapport and trust, but for enabling the practice of the *best* medicine. It is a rare health insurance policy that will adequately compensate the family physician for his or her time and expertise, yet most will fully cover extensive medical imaging and surgical procedures without question.

The typical drug ad shows a TV actor in a white laboratory coat extolling the virtues of a flashy new medicine, followed by a soothing voice in the background sliding over a drug's the drawbacks, with this final admonition: "Ask your doctor about Brand X and see if it is right for you." The implication is that this bit of knowledge gained by the viewer and brought to the busy doctor will enable an appropriate prescription—another attempt at undermining of the primary doctor's judgment. I truly admire the physician who can keep tabs on the myriad of new drugs that continually make their appearance.

Listen to Your Body

Beginning in the 1960s, whether it was for the purpose of looking good, feeling good, or being healthy, there was a great surge of interest in nutrition, exercise, and avoidance of environmental toxins. "Listen to your body" was the mantra. Don't put questionable chemicals in your body. Even little hole-in-the-wall lunch counters prepared excellent, nutritionally sound sandwiches. Exercise was the rage. Kenneth Cooper, M.D., who designed the physical testing criteria for Air Force cadets, gave us a new concept, "aerobic fitness," that motivated many to get active. Informative articles on good nutrition appeared in popular magazines. And finally, smoking was roundly condemned by everyone who didn't smoke or profit from smoking.

To its credit, the medical establishment bolstered the talk of the necessity of exercise. After President Dwight Eisenhower's heart attack in 1955, his cardiologist, Dr. Paul Dudley White, admonished his own colleagues to stop advising patients to lie in bed after a heart attack and start them on a graduated exercise program as soon as possible, beginning in the hospital itself. Dr. White was a very trim man who was often seen in a suit and tie riding his bicycle for transportation around Washington, D.C., with his "doctor bag" on board.

There are things you can do today to get healthy and stay healthy, without the need for drugs or surgery.

HEALTH UN-SURANCE

Health insurance should cover preventive and therapeutic megadoses of vitamins. It doesn't. Now, think this one over: the erectile dysfunction drug Viagra is covered by most health plans, according to its manufacturer, Pfizer Inc. Pfizer admits that Viagra may cause "heart attack, stroke, irregular heartbeat, and death" in some persons, even those without preexisting heart conditions. Compare that with the fact that high-dose vitamin E and C supplements prevent heart attack and stroke and reduce cardiovascular deaths by up to 50 percent. And still, substantially any use of vitamins is not covered by most "health" plans. I (AWS) will bet your own health "un-surance" won't even cover a daily multiple vitamin. It is much more likely to cover grandpa's access to a better sex life than to pay for vitamins for his grandchildren.

People who rely on financial assistance from the government will find that food stamps, administered by the U.S. Department of Agriculture, cannot be used to buy vitamins. Some skeptical people I've talked to think this is tantamount to conspiracy. Whether or not that is the case does not matter nearly as much as this does: Take charge of, and responsibility for, your family's health. My mother always said, "You can only spend your money in one place." Use it wisely and invest in wellness. It is cheaper in the long run.

As I said, my children never needed to take antibiotics. When we had insurance (which was rarely), it did not help us at all. My kids had their physicals at school and, economically thus vetted, they played outdoors, ate right, and took their vitamins. Insurance did not pay for any of the vitamins or the good food that kept them well.

But as for erectile dysfunction, just sign here!

WHO ARE THE QUACKS?

Let's ask George Bernard Shaw. In his great preface to an otherwise unremarkable play, *The Doctor's Dilemma* (1906), he wrote: "The distinction between a quack doctor and a qualified one is mainly that only the qualified one is authorized to sign death certificates, for which both sorts seem to have about equal occasion." Ouch. Of course, Mr. Shaw was not about to hold it at that. "Nobody supposes that doctors are less virtuous than judges; but a judge whose salary and reputation depended on whether the verdict was for plaintiff or defendant, prosecutor or prisoner, would be as little trusted as a general in the pay of the enemy."

He continues: "But just as the best carpenter or mason will resist the introduction of a machine that is likely to throw him out of work, so the doctor will resist with all his powers of persecution every advance of science that threatens his income. . . . It unluckily happens that the organization of private practitioners which we call the medical profession is coming more and more to represent, not science, but desperate and embittered anti-science.

"The only evidence that can decide a case of malpractice is expert evidence: that is, the evidence of other doctors; and every doctor will allow a colleague to decimate a whole countryside sooner that violate the bond of professional etiquette by giving him away.... All that can be said for medical popularity is that until there is a practicable alternative to blind trust in the doctor, the truth about the doctor is so terrible that we dare not face it."

Mr. Shaw was right on all counts save one: there *is* a practical alternative and there always has been—learn to do it yourself. Be your own doctor and manage your own case. Change your life and live healthier starting today. By the way, G.B. Shaw was a vegetarian, hated vaccination, and lived to be ninety-four.

In order to avoid sounding like we "bash" doctors just as the doctors "bash" us, I (RC) definitely want to tone down Shaw's comments. I will not try to defend the arrogance of a doctor who refuses to consider even a discussion of nutritional factors in disease, but we should not put *all* doctors into that category. There *are* knowledgeable, conscientious doctors ready to practice good medicine. The problem is our "health insurance care," not health care insurance. The insurance company limits what the doctor can do if he or she intends to be reimbursed financially. This allows only a little time for obtaining a medical and nutrition history, a good physical examination, and outlining a treatment plan. Shortcuts come in the form of prescriptions and referrals to specialists. Some medical schools have included nutrition science into their medical education curricula, but the positive effect won't be noticed immediately. At least for now, your best bet in finding a suitable doctor is not through a medical directory but by patient referral.

Lobbying for Unpopular Alternatives

Unorthodox medicine, unpopular research, and drugless healing have always come in for criticism by allopathic or drug-and-surgery doctors. My (AWS) feeling is that there's nothing wrong with disagreement among the health professions, because this keeps practitioners aware that there are varied approaches to wellness, not just their own. The problem arises when one school of treatment comes into political power and strongly biases the laws of the land against alternative schools of treatment.

Law sometimes is the last aspect of a country's rising consciousness to show revision. If you read your state's Medical Practice Act, you may be amazed at the strong restriction of any non-medical approach to healing. The Medical Practice Act in New York will be found under "Education" in the Consolidated Laws Service, section 6501, and is twenty-five pages in length. The Act is full of case notes and records of convictions of those who "practiced medicine without a license" including a beautician "who treated and prescribed for blemishes on the face of a patron."

"Quackery" is supposed to be harmful, and the law is there to protect us from charlatans. Not everyone knows that the original meaning of the word *charlatan* is just an unregistered health practitioner, not a health criminal. If the law is supposed to help us, how can we explain in one case that "the fact that the treatments were in some instances beneficial is wholly immaterial" to the trial of an unlicensed practitioner in New York? Because the issue is not health, but business: a state's medical practice act protects the exclusiveness of the allopathic medical doctor from competition by rendering an outsider's practice illegal. Public health has little to do with it.

But you have to make up your mind about that yourself. Don't let the medical politicians make up your mind for you, try as they may. Deciding, choosing, and verifying in your own life which health methods are truly life supporting should be restricted by no law, doctor, or attitude. This is why we must all "lobby" and call for freedom of health. Please write your lawmakers and tell them your views. It has been said that no king with his scepter wields more power than informed citizens holding pens.

TEACH YOURSELF

I (AWS) raised my children into adulthood without their ever requiring a single dose of an antibiotic, and I have Drs. Frederick R. Klenner and Lendon H. Smith to thank for it. A student came up to me one day after a lecture and placed a slim paperback into my hands, saying, "You have to read this!" The little book was Dr. Smith's *Vitamin C as a Fundamental Medicine* (since retitled *Clinical Guide to the Use of Vitamin C*). It is a digest of Dr. Klenner's medical papers, some dating from the 1940s, which had been collected, summarized, and annotated by Dr. Smith into a mere fifty-seven pages of astounding reading. Since much of Dr. Klenner's work was published in regional medical journals, his articles previously had been hard to come by.

The antibiotic and antiviral effects of megadoses of vitamin C have been largely unappreciated by the health professions. Dr. Klenner's forty years of experience successfully treating pneumonia, herpes, mononucleosis, hepatitis, multiple sclerosis, childhood illnesses, fevers, encephalitis, polio, and over twenty other diseases, all with vitamin C, is even less well known to the general public. Patients and orthodox physicians typically are amazed when they learn that Dr. Klenner employed high doses of vitamin C (350–1,000 mg per kilogram of patient body weight per day). One can only speculate how much suffering might have been avoided if doctors in the 1950s had listened to this man.

The word *doctor* is derived form the Latin word for "teacher." If your physician is a good health coach, great. If he or she is not, then you absolutely need to doctor (teach) yourself. Here is a quick way to evaluate your doctor's alternative health potential. Ask your doctor if he or she agrees with this statement: "There is a natural substitute for nearly every drug. I do not want to use nutrition and vitamin supplements along with drugs. I want to use them *instead* of drugs." If your doctor is intolerant of such a position, or simply not up to speed, you can either help fill the void or go to another doctor.

Watch One, Do One, Teach One

"That's how we learn," a surgical resident told me over three decades ago, when I (AWS) first gowned up as a student observer in the operating room. "Watch a procedure, then do it, and then teach it. Here,"

he added, "Hold that clamp like this. Yes, that's it." He had no business letting me assist with surgery, but the patient was out like a light,
and the rest of us all had masks on anyway. So, I began to learn how
to learn: watch and copy.

Interestingly enough, that's also how I learned to fly an airplane.
"Pay attention," my 275-pound, red-faced flight instructor said. "If
you get it right on the first attempt, the flight examiner won't ask you
for more." As much as I dreaded the flight test, I actually paid attention for a much stronger reason: I considered my overweight and
hypertensive instructor to be a prime candidate for a mile-high heart
attack. If he was going to die in the air, I was not about to let him
take me with him. I wanted to be able to control and land that plane
in the worst way. I was plenty motivated—I wanted to live.

Motivation is a wonderful thing. Survival is probably the most
powerful motivator there is. The breath of life is everyone's number
one concern. No one wants to sicken and die, and sick people very
much want to get well. That is why the most common use of Internet searches is for information on a disease topic.

But how else can we learn when physicians are generally so unwill-
ing to really teach us? There is only one path left to us: we'll teach
ourselves. Most doctors do not explain their trade secrets any more
than medieval guild members would show peasants how to make their
own sword, purify their own silver, or read Latin. If you made your
own sword, why have elite nobles and knights? If serfs had access to
their own silver, they would buy their freedom. If everyone could read,
history would change. And when everyone read, history did change.

Changing your present, and thereby your future, sounds even better. The goal of this book is to improve parents' abilities in self-reliant
health care. We think one way to do this is to demystify medicine of its
needlessly confusing terminology. Another way is to simultaneously
present both the validity, and the simplicity, of natural health care.
That means simplification without dumbing it down. After over thirty-
five years in the field, I am well aware that accomplishing such a goal
is no easy task. The message "change your life" is simple—but doing
so is not easy.

One of the best parts of the old *Prevention* magazine (that is, a few decades ago, when it still had J.I. Rodale's editorial teeth) was the letters sent in by readers. Such natural-health testimonials and anecdotes are all too quickly dismissed by doctors. Doctors even tend to dismiss other doctors' case reports . . . unless, of course, they like what is reported. Yet, all our teachers have said (and any kindergarten graduate knows) that this is how we learn: from others. We add it all in and think it over. As parents, surely we keep learning all the time, every day.

When you do share your health experiences with your doctor or others, I have a suggestion. Medical journal references, and quotes taken from them, add to the credibility of your reporting. Be sure to cite some scientific studies. State University of New York Professor John I. Mosher has described this in terms of baboons. Sometimes a potential rival baboon challenges the leadership of the troop's dominant male. The issue is generally decided by a form of majority vote. If more of the baboons stand behind the challenger, he takes over; if most stand behind the current leader, he remains in charge. Dr. Mosher said it is about the same with research references: try to get as many baboons as you can to back you up.

CONTROVERSY OVER VITAMIN THERAPY

Vitamin therapy is a triple threat to the medical cartel. It threatens doctors because most know practically nothing about it and cannot control it with their prescriptions. It threatens pharmaceutical companies because vitamins cannot be patented and sold at huge profits. It threatens many an old-school dietitian because the fallaciousness of the food-groups-always, supplements-just-about-never dogma will be exposed. In all three cases, it is the very success of vitamin therapy that is cause for such alarm.

The only sure way to quash the spread of vitamin therapy is to discredit those who champion it. It is the world's oldest way to stop progress: call it fraud. Attack the person, not the idea. If you dislike the singer, you'll never hear the song. A really bright dictator doesn't have to burn books; just getting people to not want to read them is sufficient.

Offbeat magicians Penn and Teller were asked what they say when someone asks how a trick is done. "Tell them," Penn said, "to go to a magician's supply shop and ask the people there. Not one of your friends will even bother to do that much research."

Good point. When I went against the grain in the colleges I taught in, no one once asked me to provide references to substantiate my views. What I knew was immaterial. In one instance, my supervising dean had been chronically and somewhat mysteriously ill for months. His doctors had no diagnosis, but immune dysfunction and chronic fatigue were suspected. This same dean admitted more than once that the vitamin information I'd given him (protocols, research papers, hints on therapy) had helped him greatly. He went so far as to assert that taking 20,000 mg of vitamin C daily was the only thing that enabled him to work at all. There was a one-pound bottle of vitamin C crystals on his desk as he sat there and dressed me down for my views.

Well, these things happen. Chinese philosopher Chaung Tsu (circa fourth century BCE) tells an old folk story: Once there was a big tree full of monkeys. They hung by their tails, they ate and they chattered, and they scurried about the tree. Along came some hunters, one of whom shot an arrow up at them. One of the monkeys casually caught the arrow, harmlessly holding it in his paw. The hunter, intrigued, shot another arrow at that monkey. The monkey caught that arrow just as effortlessly.

"This is incredible!" the hunter said to his companions. "Let's go tell the emperor!"

They immediately went to the palace and described what they had seen. Of course, the emperor wanted to see it too, so he and a dozen of his best warriors rode their horses at a gallop to the monkey tree. Things looked just as before, with monkeys chattering, eating, and scurrying about. You couldn't tell one monkey from another.

"Which monkey is the clever one?" asked the emperor.

"I can't tell, your highness," said the hunter.

"Then we'll find out. Archer, shoot an arrow at the monkeys."

The king's best marksman let an arrow fly. It was caught by the clever monkey, in his right paw.

"Another arrow," said the emperor.

This time the archer aimed straight at the clever monkey. The monkey easily caught the arrow with his left paw.

"Again," said the emperor.

The archer shot a third arrow, which the monkey caught using his right foot.

The emperor watched the monkey, hanging by his left foot, grasping three arrows, and chattering away.

"I've never seen anything like that!" exclaimed the emperor. "Now, all of you archers shoot at once."

The twelve warriors all shot arrows together and killed the monkey.

The moral? Being the clever one doesn't always make you popular! Prophets are not always appreciated in their hometowns. Innovation may be opposed, especially by those who stand to gain by squelching it. After all, where is the money in self-reliance? Sometimes, we have to say no to conformity, and sometimes we have to duck some arrows when we do. But be brave and keep looking outside the pharmaceutical medicine box.

HEALTH SELF-RELIANCE FOR FUN AND PROFIT

Back-to-nature pioneer Scott Nearing stated the following in his 1976 book *The Making of a Radical*: "The average American has no idea what good health is or how to go about obtaining it. When he feels the effects of ill health he goes to a doctor, who, like his prospective patient, knows little or nothing about health although he knows a great deal about diseases. . . . Suffering from disease we treat the results of bad living instead of learning to live a good life with its normal consequences: painless functioning of the organism. This desperately bad situation leaves it to food cranks like us to practice health and keep clear of disease and doctors."[1]

"Complementary medicine" sure sounds good. It sounds like progressive, real health-care reform, an ideal marriage of the best of the old and the new, the scientific and the holistic, the technological and the natural, the doctor and the patient. But for those of us who favor wellness self-reliance, it is a far cry from alternative health. Alternative health is different, first in the obvious way: the word *medicine* is not there, which means the medical and pharmaceutical professions are cut out. And since they don't want that, they are willing to accept some of the "natural" stuff as long as they maintain control of writing and filling prescriptions. But they will not support you when you go off on your own, to your own garden or to your local health food store or to your own library or Internet research.

If you've ever met a plumber or electrician or appliance repairman or auto mechanic who said, "Here, let me show you how to do this," then you have been singularly fortunate. Rare as this experience may be, it is infinitely more rare for health professionals to teach you exactly how to dispense with their services. An underlying assumption implicit in fee-for-service medical care is that you can't do what the doctor does, and you are a fool for thinking you can.

Decades ago, I (AWS) once was stranded out of state with all my car's radiator fluid bleeding out, staining the parking lot nicely green. It was Sunday, I could not find a mechanic who would come to the car, and I had no money for a tow or, for that matter, for an overnight stay to wait for the job to be eventually attended to. So, I pleaded with, and ultimately convinced, a gas station attendant to loan me a few tools and drop a hint about how to replace coolant hoses. This might sound like small potatoes to you, but I was a nineteen-year-old egghead and up until then had never worked under a car in my life. The prospect actually frightened me. But I learned that desperation and elbow grease will loosen even the frayed plumbing of an old Ford. I replaced the hose, filled the radiator, returned the tools, and drove away.

Not long ago, I discovered that you can call some appliance factories and, for a fee, they will walk you through the repair over the phone. Outback Australian children have been taught by radio for decades. I am convinced that doctors could do this with us, by radio for free or by phone for a fee. I've been saying for years how much I'd like to see neighborhood health instruction co-ops. Car self-repair, appliance self-repair, and health self-repair require a common attitude: "This is learnable, this is do-able, and I can learn to do it." It is a lot like being a pioneer, a homesteader on the frontier.

Consider the financial aspects of all this. What if we were determined to do without pharmaceuticals? Common assumption: certainly we can't. Health homesteader's assumption: maybe we can. The difference? The health homesteader takes back control. No longer a patient, the health homesteader gains knowledge, experience, and self-reliance, in that order. Granted, there are times when we absolutely do require a professional. But we can act to greatly reduce the frequency of those times, far beyond what we've been told.

COIK

When they returned from being stationed in the former Dutch colony of Aruba, my Navy uncle and aunt brought me a plastic model kit. I was thrilled until I opened it: it was a waterwheel-style flourmill, of all things. I do not know exactly what they were thinking, as warplanes and model cars were much more to my seven-year-old taste at the time. And what's more, the model had absolutely no instructions in English, just diagrams.

Undaunted, I got out my model glue and opened every window in the house for ventilation, just as my Dad always told me to. Then, I proceeded to assemble my multinational plastic flourmill. I did pretty well, until I came to step 11. I distinctly recall how confused I was by a part that looked like a round metal box with a red plastic tube protruding from one of its sides and a blue tube from the other. Each tube seemed to be filled with a hard shiny substance, and if you bent them, they kept their shape. The pictures indicated that the center of the round silver box was to be attached to the water wheel. The red and blue things were to be connected to something with a plus sign and a minus sign that was not included in the kit. Arrows showed that if you did this magic, the wheel somehow would turn round and round. But at that young age, I did not yet understand the concept of electricity. I simply did not know.

Today, as you read this, you might be inclined to say, "Those were wires for connecting to a battery, kid. You don't get out much, do you?" That's because it is clear to you, and it is clear because you already know it. And that is what COIK means: "Clear Only If Known." But a minute ago, you knew as much about what COIK stood for as I once knew about electricity.

This story illustrates two important points. First, some people simply are not aware; they do not know what to do. There is such a thing as ignorance. Among professionals, it is sometimes masked by a haughty attitude. For most folks, it is innocent. Second, language remains a big barrier in international relations, model building, and health care. Complex Latin medical terms and fancy technical words are stumbling blocks for many people who seek to become their own doctor.

You can sidestep this problem with a medical dictionary or an Internet search. I recommend, and regularly use, the *Merck Manual* when I have to look up a term. (Your library has one and it is also available online.) And when you use it, don't be bashful; remember what Albert Einstein supposedly said when asked some trivial factual detail: "I don't know." The questioner was flabbergasted at such an answer from such a man, but Einstein allegedly merely replied, "Why should I clutter my head with things I can look up?"

SUMMARY

When you take more responsibility for your family's health care, you are that much less a patient and that much more a parent. Look into natural alternatives and see for yourself. Do not hesitate to consider non-medical, non-pharmaceutical resources. "Have no respect for the authority of others," said philosopher Bertrand Russell, "for there are always contrary authorities to be found." As you read more about nutritional medicine, you strengthen your position when you do need to go to the doctor. Knowledge is power and, more important, your added health knowledge means healthier children.

CHAPTER 3

THE TRUTH ABOUT ANTIBIOTICS AND IMMUNIZATIONS

*"For every drug that benefits a patient, there is a
natural substance that can achieve the same effect."*
—CARL C. PFEIFFER, M.D., PH.D.

Two of the so-called successes of allopathic medicine are antibiotics and vaccinations, which have proven remarkably effective in some cases. However, overuse and questionable applications of these medicines have cast a shadow over them. Natural alternatives to boost immune function, continually downplayed by conventional practitioners and the pharmaceutical companies, may prove more effective and safer in the long run.

"WEAPONS OF MASS DESTRUCTION" AGAINST BACTERIA

The appearance of antibiotics, the "weapons of mass destruction" against bacteria responsible for infectious diseases, was preceded by an explosion of knowledge of the target. Near the end of the nineteenth century, two amazing men, pioneers in the science of bacteriology, contributed mightily to this discipline.

Prussian-born scientist Robert Koch (1843–1910) formed his postulate that a specific disease is caused by a specific bacterium. He is noted for isolating the bacteria that cause tuberculosis and cholera. His students isolated the respective organisms responsible for anthrax, diphtheria, typhoid, pneumonia, gonorrhea, meningitis (the common form), leprosy, bubonic plague, tetanus, and syphilis. It is truly amazing that he could imagine such diverse organisms as hard-shelled endospores from the soil, which "spontaneously" change to the causative agent of anthrax, and wiggly (under the microscope) spirochetes, the agent of syphilis, as causes of disease. Dr. Koch developed tools of investigation that are still in use: the blood-agar plates (and petri dishes) for growing bacteria for diagnostic purposes and further study.

German scientist Paul Ehrlich (1854–1915) was called to work with Dr. Koch in the Prussian Institute for Infectious Diseases in 1891. While learning all they could of these pathogens, Dr. Ehrlich's niche was oriented to finding "chemo" agents that would kill the pathogens. Prior to his time the only anti-syphilitic agents were inorganic mercury compounds. Just by experimenting with various agents in the petri dish, his staff developed an organic arsenical agent marketed as "Salvarsan." In 1912, a new and improved chemical agent, named Neosalvarasan, was much easier to administer than the former but was slightly less effective. In their day, each of these arsphenamine drugs was considered to be a "magic bullet" for the treatment of syphilis. We moderns do not have high regard for either mercury or arsenic, but the alternative of raging madness, then death, from tertiary syphilis would even today be considered unacceptable. A nineteenth-century German equivalent of our Centers for Disease Control might also state, "effectiveness outweighs potential risk." At any rate, this was *the* treatment of syphilis until the appearance of penicillin in the 1940s.

During the interim, sulfa (or sulpha) drugs had their share of the spotlight in bacterial disease treatment. In the 1930s, it was discovered that sulfanilamide, a component of a dye, provided effective treatment for streptococcal infections. It worked in the body but not in the test tube. The reason for this discrepancy was discovered in 1940. Sulfanilamide inhibits the action of para-aminobenzoic acid, which bacteria need to make folic acid, a vitamin that has many vital functions and is essential for life. As with "chemo" for cancer, the more rapidly growing cells are hit the hardest. Many derivatives of sulfanilamide were developed and put on the market and were somewhat effective in the treatment of other "coccal" organisms: *Staphylococcus* and *Pneumococcus*. In a relatively short time, though, bacterial resistance to sulfas developed. The basic mechanism of creating a folic acid deficiency in the bacterium many times trickled over to unacceptable side effects in the host.

Antibiotic is the term given to a chemical substance derived from one organism that is destructive to another organism. In the case of penicillin, a mold, *Penicillium notatum,* was the progenitor. I (RC) always thrilled to the drama of British bacteriologist Alexander Fleming (1881–1955) accidentally stumbling upon the discovery of colonies of *Staphylococcus aureus,* growing in a Petri dish of growth medium in his laboratory, being annihilated by something from a growth of an adjacent contaminant mold. Whether or not the mold was an unwelcome contaminant was not the issue. Being a bacteriologist, Fleming knew of the use of certain molds, even in ancient Chinese medicine, for treating pus-forming infections. There was a good deal of research in the 1890s directed to studying the role of molds in fighting infection. He understood that there had to be a substance in the mold that "cleared" the plate of the *Staphylococcus.* Next, he grew the mold and identified it. He tested a pure *Penicillium* culture on many different bacterial cultures and found the killing effect. That magical substance, from then on, was simply called penicillin.

After the discovery of the substance and its great potential, the trick was to find methods that would vastly increase production of the mold. Teaming up with interested parties in the United States, Fleming found methods that increased yields ten times over, creating

"Antibiotic resistance comes mainly because of inappropriate or improper use of antibiotics by physicians. Some 150 million prescriptions are written annually in this country. And 60 percent of them—that translates to 90 million prescriptions—are for antibiotics. Of those, 50 million are absolutely unnecessary or inappropriate."

—Dr. Philip Tierno, director of clinical microbiology and diagnostic immunology at New York University Medical Center enough to be used in designed clinical trials. Progressive success in production yielded enough penicillin to be used in 1943 for U.S. soldiers wounded in the D-Day invasion. In 1945, even though I (RC) had not realized it at the time, I had entered the ground floor of the antibiotic revolution.

Antibiotics and Navy Hospital Corpsman Campbell

With the World War Two draft still in place during my last year of high school, I chose to go into the Navy Hospital Corps when I was to be called up. Oddly enough, the "call" came on August 15, 1945, the day the Japanese surrendered. I had been warned during my Navy physical examination that the Japanese were using the Red Cross insignia on corpsmen's uniforms for target practice. The call was the epitome of mixed emotions: thankfulness for not being made a target; sadness for having to give up my carefree life. Corpsmen were given grave responsibilities, either on board ship or in land-based hospitals. After a few weeks of school, I was assigned to duty at the Marine Corps Boot Camp at Camp Pendleton, California.

Now, my education truly began. Marines from overseas flooded in to be made ready for discharge from the service. Unfortunately for many, sexually transmitted diseases had to be treated and cured. Prophylactic use of a mercury ointment hadn't been effective and sulfa drugs were not working, but penicillin did work. There was no oral form of penicillin, not even a long-acting intra-muscular form, only a water-soluble form that was given every six hours for a two-day course of treatment. Here I was, a kid barely out of high school, armed with a syringe with a huge needle attached, ready to deal with these battle-hardened Marines. Also, I was glad the shots were for them and not for me. To my credit, I developed a shot-giving technique that disguised the pain of the procedure: I slapped them on one cheek and quickly plunged the needle into the other. Success was confirmed if the recipient asked, "Did you give it yet, doc?"

The "honeymoon" period for this wonder drug was less than ten years. Penicillin cured many terrible diseases attributed to streptococcal, staphylococcal, or pneumococcal (the common cause of pneumonia) infections. Persons afflicted with staph-caused boils, even if they were on a long-term basis, were rid of the problem after a single shot. Strep throat (usually called tonsillitis) was readily cured. Consequently, it was believed that rheumatic fever, a reaction to a previous strep infection, could be eliminated if sore throats were appropriately treated. I am not sure that penicillin's effectiveness with sexually transmitted diseases sent the right signal, but initially it was a very successful treatment.

THE PROBLEM OF ANTIBIOTIC RESISTANCE

My first encounter with the problem of antibiotic failure hit me forcibly. In 1956, while I was in residency training at Los Angeles Children's Hospital, my wife gave birth to our second daughter in Hollywood Presbyterian Hospital across the street. This was the hospital of the "stars" so, of course, the very highest standards of care prevailed. Delivery went well, but a few days later, we noticed the baby having difficulty breathing, and she was admitted to Children's Hospital. She was diagnosed with pneumonia and started on a regimen of I.M. (intramuscular) penicillin and streptomycin, the standard treatment for a newborn with pneumonia. Breathing became more labored, and a chest x-ray was repeated. Her lungs looked like Swiss cheese—numerous air cells, partially filled with fluid, were seen throughout both lungs. A blood culture was done, revealing hemolytic *Staphylococcus aureus*. "Hemolytic" refers to the colony of the bacterium eating a clear spot out of the blood-containing growth medium.

So, this lowly resident doctor challenged the medical director of the hospital to switch the antibiotic treatment. The alternative proved to be lifesaving for our baby but was fraught with serious side effects for some, leading to it eventually being taken off the market. Subsequently, many more cases of "cystic" pneumonia were admitted to this hospital. Many of these patients went on to develop life-threatening pneumothorax, which is a blow-out of one or more of the cysts, creating free air in the chest cavity that could collapse a lung. Our daughter was the only one of many with a positive blood culture for "staph" who didn't suffer a pneumothorax.

This ordinary germ had become extraordinary: penicillin did not do what it was expected to do because the bacteria had developed antibiotic resistance. Pharmaceutical companies had an urgent job to do. They quickly had to develop a new weapon to defeat this organism, but they also had to educate physicians and the public concerning the threat. No longer should such a potent tool as an antibiotic be prescribed with little forethought. Unfortunately, this resolve did not prevail. It was as if the medical community could not be awakened out of its pleasant dream.

Another mold-derived antibiotic, erythromycin, was developed that was effective for treatment of the "cocci," and still is for some. A next-generation of penicillin, methicillin, was developed specifically for treatment of resistant "staph," but many strains of the bacterium have now become methicillin resistant. Soon, other organisms became resistant to the antibiotics that had once been effective, and whole new classes of antibiotics were developed, many of them derived from other molds. They all met similar fates for similar reasons, plus some were fraught with terrible side effects, such as deafness in newborns or kidney damage. Effectiveness can go from good, to so-so, to null on an unpredictable time schedule.

As each new antibiotic was developed, the experts in the field admonished doctors to prevent bacterial antibiotic resistance by:

- Using the appropriate antibiotic for a specified *bacterial* infection. Antibiotics are useless against viruses.

- Using the newly developed antibiotic only when the old ones are no longer effective. This can be enhanced by checking with the local hospital laboratory to see what pathologic strains are in the community and from the results of sensitivity tests.

- Reserving at least one newly developed antibiotic for exclusive inpatient hospital use rather than widely prescribing it.

- Making sure patients take the full course of antibiotic to prevent the emergence of tougher residual bacteria that would require higher doses in the future.

- Explaining to patients that antibiotics never were a "cure-all" for fever or viral infections and that pharmaceutical companies may not be able to stay one step ahead with the development of new antibiotics if these steps are not taken.

These directives have not been completely heeded. It is currently estimated that 47 percent of antibiotic prescriptions are "inappropriate." By pharmaceutical companies blitzing doctors about the latest antibiotic, and media attention along the same lines, we still have many who think that prescribing a new antibiotic is going to a *stronger* antibiotic. If the change results in effective treatment, strength has nothing to do with it. *Appropriateness* has everything to do with it. Failing to honestly educate the public about the necessity of thoughtful use of these great tools has put enormous pressure on doctors to yield to their patients' desire rather than providing the "best medicine."

For years, there had been one "ace in the hole" for treating the resistant "coccal" infections, vancomycin, reserved strictly for hospital use when sensitivity tests found nearly all other antibiotics were ineffective for that patient's particular disease-causing bacterium. Then, even vancomycin-resistant bacteria began emerging, giving rise to "superbugs" and "flesh-eating strep or staph," leaving us with few weapons to combat this serious problem. Other drugs "of last resort" have replaced vancomycin.

The problem is compounded when a patient from one area enters a distant hospital (a tertiary center) suitable for the patient's special needs. Bacteria peculiar to the locale of that hospital can ride piggyback on patients discharged to their home communities. These bacteria may not cause overt disease, but they can survive in a carrier. Nevertheless, bad bugs have started new homes.

OVERUSE OF ANTIBIOTICS IN ANIMAL HUSBANDRY

Rather than resigning ourselves to a fate something akin to a horror movie, let's get serious about implementing control that we know will help. Doctors should actually treat antibiotics with respect by follow-

ANTIBIOTICS IN FEED, CATTLE, AND HUMANS

Howard Lyman, a raised-to-graze, fourth-generation dairy farmer and cattle rancher, is that arch-heretic of animal husbandry: he's a vegan. Lyman and his expert collaborator, Glen Merzer, wrote *Mad Cowboy: Plain Truth from the Cattle Rancher Who Won't Eat Meat,*[1] an in-your-face book full of meat-busting facts. This book really homes in on the range.

Lyman writes that slaughterhouse quality control, such as it is, simply is not working. "About 80 percent of food poisonings come from meat," Lyman states. "Approximately 30 percent of chicken consumed in America is contaminated with salmonella, and 70–90 percent with another deadly pathogen, *Campylobacter*." In America, contaminated chicken kills over 1,000 people annually and sickens perhaps 80 million more. Oversight and inspection by the U.S. Department of Agriculture and the Food and Drug Administration is so lax because they "can generally be counted on to behave not like public servants but like hired hands of the meat and dairy industries." The government inspects only one out of every 250,000 carcasses.

Lyman also claims that most meat is contaminated with carcinogens such as dioxins (halogenated hydrocarbons) and DDT. Cattle feed is higher in pesticides than crops grown directly for human consumption. A *New England Journal of Medicine* study found that the breast milk of vegetarian women had only 1–2 percent of the national average of pesticide contamination.[2]

A young Mr. Lyman knew nothing of all this. Doing farm chores at age five, castrating calves at age ten, and paying his way through agricultural college with poker winnings, he was determined to make a success of feedlot farming. And he did, lacing the feed of his 7,000 steers with antibiotics, diethylstilbesterol (DES), and an array of other "suspect" drugs purchased in quantity just before they were banned. It was a rough life, especially for the cattle. "The flies can get so thick they actually threaten a cow's ability to breathe," he writes. "Every morning I would fill up a fly fogger with insecticide and spray great clouds of it over the whole operation." In following such practices, dangerous as they are to animals, farmer, and the public, Lyman's cattle operation was not unusual.

Lyman's book includes an account of his ever-increasing health problems as a cattleman, which finally forced his reconsideration of the ethics and the consequences of his livelihood. Even after serious spine surgery, a meat-fed Lyman "weighed 350 pounds, my cholesterol was over 300, my blood pressure was off the charts, and I was getting nosebleeds," in addition to eyesight problems. His response was to change his entire life: he switched to organic farming and became a vegetarian. "Within a year of eating no meat, my health problems all started to go away. Everything revolved around the fork," Lyman asserts. "Since I became a vegetarian eight years ago, I have lost 130 pounds steadily, gradually, and without trying. I never gained any of the weight back, and never felt hungry. I never went on a diet, never counted my calories. I simply stopped eating animal products. My cholesterol count declined from 300 to 140, my blood pressure went from dangerously high levels to normal ones, and my energy levels increased."

We should not attribute all the improvement in health and laboratory reports just to the absence of meat in his diet, because he effectively improved his diet across the board. The vegetarian diet is full of healthful nutrients; most notable is the absence of so-called antinutrients, such as sugar and junk food. In 1996, Lyman along with Oprah Winfrey were sued for "food disparagement" by a group of Texas cattlemen. In 1998, he won the lawsuit, and the result was *Mad Cowboy*.

ing the outline described above. Stop practices that we know result in pathologic strains of *E. coli*, *Salmonella*, and *Campylobacter* entering our food chain. Specifically, we need to stop the dangerous ways we raise commercial food animals. In the case of cattle, our agriculture authorities recommended antibiotics as part of the standard of animal husbandry. The idea was that giving antibiotics to young, healthy animals would prevent energy-robbing infections, thus acting as a growth stimulant.

Incredibly, as early as 1963, the antibiotics used for this practice—penicillin, streptomycin, erythromycin—were ones currently being used for treating human infections. Whether or not animals showed signs of the bacterial infections that these drugs were designed to treat, their intestinal flora now included resistant strains of these bacteria. As the problem was recognized, the same hunt for effective antibiotics was undertaken in animals as it was for humans. Animals shipped many miles, then put into a crowded feedlot, are stressed, putting an added burden on their immune systems. Living in this crowded cesspool encourages massive cross-infection. Slaughterhouses and meat packing facilities aren't much better, so it is easy to see how pathogenic bacteria get into the food chain.

There are many different strains of *Salmonella*, the worst of which are not spread by animals. But the rest are (or via contaminated water), arriving in about every edible substance. We are constantly reminded of food contamination by this organism as a cause of severe intestinal upset. The role of undercooked beef in *E. coli* 0157:H7 outbreaks can cause bloody diarrhea and occasionally life-threatening kidney failure. Chickens can carry another serious pathogen, *Campylobacter*, in their intestinal tracts, which can cause a severe illness starting with flu-like symptoms of fever, headache, muscle aches, then a watery, sometimes bloody diarrhea, accompanied with severe abdominal cramps.

Another spin-off from adding antibiotics to animal feed is the problem of antibiotic-resistant bacterial strains, including "supergerms," residing in the animal's gut. The bacteria are spewed onto the ground. From there, either from rainfall or irrigation, they can run off into a body of water—water that could irrigate the spinach you eat. Instead of hiring more food inspectors, we need laws to stop the addition of antibiotics to animal feed. The sad part of this story is our failure to learn from past experiences. Antibiotics in the fluoroquinolone class were used in chicken feed. Currently, these antibiotics, the big guns for the "superbugs," are no longer useful for fighting *Salmonella* or *Campylobacter* infections. The government health authorities recognize the problem, but don't hold your breath waiting for the enactment of a solution. The food industries are too powerful.

THE PROPER USE OF ANTIBIOTICS

The more courses of antibiotic treatment taken, the greater the likelihood of encountering a resistant strain. Antibiotics kill not only enemy bacteria but bacterial allies (friendly bacteria), too. It is well documented that people who have recently undergone a course of antibiotic treatment are more susceptible to having a resistant organism fill the void. Maintaining a higher concentration of "good" bacteria in the intestinal tract reduces the chance of "bad" bacteria getting a foothold, for the good and the bad are competing for the same nutrients. When the balance of the intestinal flora is upset, ordinary harmless bacteria can become bacterial "terrorists." Increasing the numbers of good bacteria is most easily done by adding cultures of *Lactobacilli* of various types (called probiotics, the most popular being acidophilus) to milk, as in yogurt or buttermilk. The authors prefer whole-milk yogurt to low-fat, because butter fat encourages the growth of these beneficial bacteria. Cultured buttermilk can be a useful staple in the diet once a taste for it is acquired.

We also need to do everything we can to boost the immune system's response to these assaults by "bad" bacteria. In general, the best boost comes from healthful living. Specifically for the problem of bacterial antibiotic resistance, consider:

- Working with your doctor to take an antibiotic only when absolutely necessary. If your doctor seems quick to prescribe, don't hesitate to speak up, say what you know, and seek his or her advice. Withholding antibiotic treatment might necessitate another quick assessment a few days later to make certain that doing without was safe. Unfavorable and unpredictable changes in the course of the illness warrant reporting and possibly another look.

- Carefully delineating the condition. Are the signs and symptoms—such as fever, nasal congestion, sore throat, trouble breathing, and heavy sinus drainage—due to an antibiotic-treatable bacterial infection? Or are they the result of a viral infection or allergy? If this sort of illness happens frequently, begin a search for the reason.

- Working more on building good health by taking vitamin D to boost your immune system along with a general vitamin-mineral supplement regimen. If you are not already doing so, add yogurt or buttermilk to your daily diet. A dash of honey or maple syrup does wonders for yogurt's acceptability and enjoyment.

- Not waiting for perfect food safety inspection, because you are going to have one long wait. In the meantime, follow the admonition to cook meat at higher temperatures. Better yet, purchase organic or grass-fed beef and range-free chicken.

- Increasing your intake of yogurt and/or probiotic supplements at the onset of any course of antibiotics, since some degree of intestinal upset is very likely.

- Taking vitamin C. In the case of antibiotic-induced diarrhea, 1,000 mg of vitamin C,three times a day, should not influence the intensity of the diarrhea. During the duration of the intestinal upset, the diet should include a water-soluble fiber source, like pectins from apples (or a commercial source) and bananas, all useful aids for reducing the severity of diarrhea.

THE VACCINATION PATHWAY: IMMUNIZATIONS AND STILL MORE IMMUNIZATIONS

When I (AWS) was a boy in the early 1960s, measles was a free ticket for two weeks off from school. Mumps, at least in the mirror, was kind of funny. And chicken pox? The worst thing about it was the name. All these illnesses were "cured" by doing nothing but staying home, eating soup until it practically came out of our noses, and watching game shows such as "Concentration," "Password," and "To Tell the Truth."

Are kids today missing out on all this? Now that there is a vaccination for everything, I do not think absenteeism is any lower than when I went to school, and it may be higher. In fact, I think attempts at artificial immunity have denied children their birthright to a rough-and-tough natural immunity. Today's kids (and tomorrow's adults) are the weaker for it.

Real immunity does not come out of a needle. The recent and spectacular failure of massive flu vaccination illustrates this. Plus, you simply cannot vaccinate everyone for everything: there are too many viruses, and they are differentiating all the time. A strong, general-purpose immune system is a necessary defense and preparation against a world of ever-new, ever-changing viruses. You need to temper the steel before you use the sword.

Trying to exist in a vaccination-blown bubble is futile. Speaking as an experienced parent and a teacher who has taught at every grade level, I think vaccinations fail to confer adequate protection. I do not think they ever did, and I do not think they do now. In a 2003 whooping cough epidemic near New York City, over 80 percent of those with the disease had been vaccinated against it (forty-four of fifty-four cases of whooping cough were in vaccinated persons).[3]

The state of New York requires some three dozen vaccinations for a baby before it is even two years old.[4] New York, and most likely your state too, obediently follows the dictates of the American Academy of Pediatrics and the American Academy of Family Physicians. Unfortunately, those two organizations are voices of authority for health insurance companies that determine how health-care providers are reimbursed. Many physicians have blind faith in these organizations and do not give enough thought to weighing advantages versus disadvantages of individual antibiotics or vaccinations. But compared to their overpowering emphasis on vaccination, and on patent drugs when immunization fails, these doctors largely ignore vitamin supplements as prevention and especially as treatment.

In the end, it's not about whether you get sick, it's about how you get well. Whether you get shots or not, I think the primary concern should be to make children's bodies strong so they can fight off disease. We do this with good food, routine supplements, and lots of vitamin C. If and when children do get sick, they will recover rapidly and without complications. Although my children were raised with vitamin supplements and a natural diet, they sometimes did get sick (not nearly as often as the neighbors' kids, however). No need to panic! Sickness happens, and the body is designed to heal. The best way to a strong immune system is through optimum nutrition and ample vitamin supplementation.

INFLUENZA VACCINE

Most literate souls who survived the 2009 influenza epidemic have some inkling of the severity of the 1918 "Spanish influenza" epidemic. It started when the "Great War" (World War One) and its participants were winding down. People's immune systems were already stressed from the drawbacks of war—disease, fatigue, poor diets, and mental stress. From what we know about viruses rearranging their genetic material to form "novel" strains that bypass the effects of herd immunity, it appears that a new, virulent strain of swine influenza was the culprit. Herd immunity comes from many people having developed antibodies and gaining partial protection to similar strains in the past. If the new virus is truly novel, there is not even partial protection but rather a great potential for a far-reaching pandemic.

Another reason why the Spanish flu was often referred to during the 2009 epidemic was that both directly attacked the lungs in those of a younger age group than usual. Secondary bacterial infection due to influenza is the most common cause of complications, but here we had young patients, who don't seem particularly ill, suddenly being found in real respiratory distress—their lungs literally filling with fluids and debris. Even though in 1918 there was no concept of "virus," this similarity is due to DNA components of influenza virus subtypes recombining to form the novel strain. In the 2009 epidemic, there were four subtypes of H1N1 involved but somehow "swine" won the title.

The effects of the Spanish flu were striking and fearsome: a fifth of the world population was infected, and an estimated 675,000 Americans died (ten times the numbers of lives lost in the war). In the worldwide population, as many soldiers died from influenza as from combat. All this horrible knowledge should be enough to promote near hysteria. It certainly got authorities such as World Health Organization (WHO) and the U.S. Centers for Disease Control and Prevention (CDC) activated. When dire predictions were not being fulfilled, these authoritative bodies fanned fears by reminding the public of the 1918 flu pandemic. Even in a "normal" influenza year, some element of fear promotion is used because it is effective.

VITAMIN D VS. THE FLU BUG

Vitamin D has known antiviral properties and has been directly associated with fighting influenza in a recent scientific review.[5] Extensive evidence, supported by recent epidemiological studies,shows that vitamin D serves as an important regulator of immune system responses.[6] Vitamin D has even been part of a supplement combination proven effective against HIV in a recent double-blind trial.[7]

During a viral infection, the body can draw on stored vitamin D to supply the increased needs of the immune system. The depleted supplies of vitamin D are quickly replenished with doses of 4,000 to 10,000 IU per day for a few days. Due to biochemical individuality, we recommend vitamin D blood testing as a routine part of a yearly physical exam.

As a county health officer, I (RC) was responsible for seeing that our citizens, particularly the older ones, were adequately prepared for the winter's expected influenza epidemic. The staff set up clinics at senior centers, with vaccine shots given after a good noon meal and conversation about "cholesterol counts" and other medical tests. The shots were a good way to keep in touch, and I was convinced of the necessity of flu vaccination. I believed what I read in my medical literature. When many complained that they got the flu after the shot, I dismissed it by saying that they were probably coming down with another virus at that time.

After all the buildup in 1976 about the dangerous swine flu—including the mention of an anticipated 30,000 deaths each year from influenza—I figured that a little fear-mongering would be effective in getting people to be immunized. After the expected epidemic was underway, one acquaintance, a man of about forty and formerly in good health, became a victim of Guillain-Barré syndrome following the flu shot. Later, there was another case. We had physicians throughout the county report infectious or unusual diseases each week, but I can't be sure that there were not other unreported cases. There were many other people who suffered severe respiratory problems that did not appear to be due to the usual secondary bacterial pneumonia. We now know this fits the pattern of other swine flu epidemics.

My attitude changed after that. The vaccine is supposed to prevent disease, not cause it. We had been told of the wonders of medical science and how scientists can go to foreign lands, isolate a strain of influenza vaccine that had caused disease, bring it to our shores, and design a vaccine for the oncoming season. The vaccine usually had two different influenza A strains and one B strain. The authorities never admitted that the vaccine missed the mark that year, but I noticed that the unvaccinated in those years were as well off as the vaccinated. So, why, the following year, had the death from influenza been the same 30,000? In a "normal" flu year, people rarely die from influenza but rather from secondary bacterial infections. The victims are usually older or have chronic illnesses, poor nutrition, and other lifestyle excesses or deficiencies, which create a poorly functioning immune system and make them predisposed to complications. These folks are singled out as those who particularly require vaccination protection. However, to my knowledge, there are no good controlled studies to confirm efficacy.

My skepticism increased after learning that vaccine producers are protected from financial loss once their product gains government sanction. When in compliance with safety and manufacturing standards, a company is licensed to produce an influenza vaccine as fast as it can, with the guarantee that it will suffer no financial loss if there is a surplus. An oversupply is rare. For many years, a last-minute mutation of the endemic virus is discovered, necessitating re-tooling and perhaps quickly qualifying another manufacturer to fill the need.

At these times, there is an attempt to downplay the urgency by telling us that the epidemic might hit later than anticipated and that, if given too early, the vaccine's benefit can diminish before the epidemic peaks. In the 2009 epidemic, by the time the vaccine supply was adequate, the epidemic had dissipated. Vaccine, then, was shamelessly hawked so that neither the manufacturers nor the government would be stuck with the bill.

Looking at past history with a new strain of swine flu, one can accept some justifiable worry on the part of authorities. Perhaps some motivation for action prompted by a bit of fear is needed. But even though the epidemic was dying out, I became truly disillusioned by the hype manipulation used by WHO and the CDC.

Another difficulty for the authorities comes from trying to sell the medical community and the public on the use of influenza medications, to be used either for treatment or prophylaxis. One shortcoming of the most popular flu medication, Tamiflu, is that the medicine has to be tuned to the specific strain of virus and might not match. It reduces the noticeable signs and symptoms of influenza by 1.3 days in the general population and 1 day for geriatric patients. My recollection of a typical bout of influenza includes about four or more days of racking cough, which makes a terrible headache worse, and aching all over. After the fever breaks, low body temperature matches very low spirits for as long as two weeks, while aches gradually subside. For me, only one day less of acute symptoms is not worth it. In 2009, British authorities disallowed the use of anti-flu drugs for children, stating that the benefits do not outweigh the harmful effects. There have been few or no studies of prophylactic efficacy in this country.

What we don't honestly know is how effective influenza immunization truly is. I don't see any studies on the horizon that are going to prove effectiveness of influenza vaccines. I do know that immune function can be improved dramatically with measures given in this book. Let's hope for some honest evaluation—we have been snowed long enough. Just as we don't need an antibiotic for every infectious disease, we can't find a vaccine for every communicable disease. The real answer is to focus on prevention and immune system health. You can afford to be bold when you have seen for yourself that these health measures work. Like everything else in my evolution, I naively trusted what I was taught only to become a true skeptic. Here's how to overcome your child's doctor's insistence on a flu shot: "Just say no!"

VITAMIN A FIGHTS MEASLES

Let's consider measles and vitamin A supplementation. The United Nations Children's Fund (UNICEF) states, "In three separate trials of children hospitalized with measles—one as early as 1932—deaths among children given high-dose vitamin A supplements were significantly lower than among children not supplemented. The consistent results suggest that a change in vitamin A status can rapidly alter basic physiological functions concerned with cellular repair and resistance to infection, thereby saving lives."[8] Note that the therapy is described as both "supplemental" and "high dose." And the trials did not have just some minor effect—they reduced deaths among these children.

Unlike finicky, vegetable-dodging children like I (AWS) was at age five, Third World children commonly do not have the luxury of good food to refuse. The answer is to teach all families in developing nations to grow their own vegetables and provide them with the land they need to do it. While vegetables are the ideal vitamin A source, the fact is that supplementation is cheaper. A malnourished child at risk of actually dying from measles constitutes an emergency. It is time to open a bottle of vitamin A—you cannot wait for the carrots to come up in the spring.

Vitamin A deficiency kills more children than the half a million it blinds. Over the past twenty years, many studies have implicated levels of vitamin A as an important determinant of health. Vitamin A intervention programs may be one of the most cost-effective health strategies in all of medicine. Women should be careful to avoid excess intake of the oil form of vitamin A in pregnancy. The good news is that carotenes from vegetable food sources are safe at all doses. Carotenes are made into vitamin A only as the body requires it.

VITAMIN C AND POLIO

Did you know that vitamin C (ascorbic acid) was shown to destroy polio viruses over seventy-five years ago?[9] The therapeutic use of tens of thousands of milligrams of vitamin C per day may be the most unacknowledged successful research in medicine. High doses were advocated immediately after ascorbic acid was isolated by Albert Szent-Györgyi, M.D., Ph.D. (1893–1986). Dr. Szent-Gyorgyi received the Nobel Prize for his ascorbate-related work in 1937.

At the turn of the 1960s, when all of us in first grade were told that we were to be vaccinated against polio, I (AWS) didn't want to go near school that day. Regardless of my fear of needles, I had no choice in the matter. So, I braced up, got in line, and marched down the tiled hallway to meet my fate. When I got to the school nurse's office, I was astounded to be handed a lump of sugar with a drop of something soaking into it. I was told to eat it. I did, then I was told I could go. Escape without a shot? What a fantastic turn of events! Life could begin anew.

In time, my classmates and I would all learn the name of our pain-less benefactor, Albert Sabin, M.D. With more time, I would find that his live oral vaccine had become the leading *cause* of polio in the U.S. What surprised me most was that the strongest criticism originated from the most eminent of sources: the other polio hero, Jonas Salk, M.D. On September 24, 1976, the *Washington Post* reported Dr. Salk's assertion that the Sabin live oral virus vaccine had been the "principal if not sole cause" of every reported polio case in the United States since 1961.[10]

In 1996, one year after Dr. Salk died, the U.S. Centers for Disease Control (CDC) began a turn-away from the oral live vaccine and rec-ommended killed virus injections for the first two rounds of infant polio immunization. By 2000, the CDC stated that "to eliminate the risk for vaccine-associated paralytic poliomyelitis, an all-injected polio virus schedule is recommended for routine childhood vaccina-tion in the United States."[11] Thus, only after two decades had passed would orthodoxy take heed of the cautionary words of Dr. Salk, the man credited with creating the first polio vaccination.

From Fame to Ascorbate to Obscurity

Drs. Sabin and Salk had media visibility, a professional rivalry, and a personal animosity spanning decades. Everyone today knows their names. By contrast, the public and orthodox medicine have yet to pay proper attention to the work of Claus W. Jungeblut, M.D. (1898–1976). Dr. Jungeblut received his M.D. from the University of Bern in 1921 and then conducted research at the Robert Koch Institute in Berlin. After employment as a bacteriologist for the New York State Department of Health from 1923 until 1927, he became Associate Professor at Stanford University and then joined the faculty at the Columbia University College of Physicians and Surgeons until his retirement in 1962.

While revisionist history of the fight against polio has generally downplayed Dr. Jungeblut's contribution to the crusade, it has sidestepped his most important discovery: that ascorbate is both prevention and cure for polio. Dr. Jungeblut first published this idea in 1935.[12] His research on ascorbate extended well beyond the topic of polio—he also showed that vitamin C inactivated diphtheria and tetanus toxins.[13]

Unlike oral polio vaccination, vitamin C has never caused polio. Yet, how many people know vitamin C has been shown to prevent and cure poliomyelitis? It was never really a secret. In September 1939, *Time* magazine reported, "Last week, at the Manhattan meeting of the International Congress for Microbiology, two new clues turned up. (One is) vitamin C."[14] The article describes how Dr. Jungeblut, while studying statistics of the 1938 Australian polio epidemic, deduced that low vitamin C status was associated with the disease. After that, Dr. Jungeblut is rarely highlighted by the popular or professional media.

Whatever Happened to Ascorbate Therapy for Polio?

When discussion about poliomyelitis turns toward megascorbate prophylaxis and treatment, there is no more frequent rejoinder than this: "If vitamin C therapy were so good, all doctors would be using it."

In his book *The Healing Factor,* Irwin Stone, Ph.D., explains why they're not: "The application of ascorbic acid in the treatment of poliomyelitis is an incredible story of high hopes that end in disappointment. . . . Within two years after the discovery of ascorbic acid, Jungeblut showed that ascorbic acid would inactivate the virus of poliomyelitis. Thus, at this early date it was established that ascorbic acid had the potential of being a wide-spectrum antiviral agent. Here was a new 'magic bullet' that was effective against a wide variety of viruses and was known to be completely harmless. . . . Sabin, attempting to reproduce Jungeblut's work on monkeys, failed to obtain these partially successful results. It may be easy for us to look back now and say that the size and the frequency of the dosages were insufficient to maintain high levels of ascorbic acid in the blood during the incubation of the disease. The upshot was that the negative findings of Sabin effectively stifled further research in this field for a decade."[15]

Since 1939, medical experts were certain that vitamin C was not effective against polio. Dr. Sabin's research, they thought, had demonstrated conclusively that vitamin C had no value in combating polio viruses. Frederick Klenner, M.D., has stated that there was a simple reason for Dr. Sabin's well-reported failures: the dosage was far too low. "One of the most unfortunate mistakes in all of the research on poliomyelitis was Sabin's unscientific attempt to confirm Jungeblut's work with vitamin C against the polio virus in monkeys. Jungeblut in infecting his rhesus monkeys used the mild 'droplet method' and then administered vitamin C by needle in varying amounts up 400 mg/day. On the other hand, Sabin, in infecting his monkeys did not follow the procedure given by Jungeblut whose experiments he was attempting to repeat, but instead employed a more forceful method of inoculation which obviously resulted in sickness of maximum severity. Sabin further refused to follow Jungeblut's suggestion as to the dose of vitamin C to be used. By Sabin's actual report the amount given was rarely more than 35 percent of that used by his associate. . . . Yet on the basis of Sabin's work the negative value of vitamin C in the treatment of virus diseases has been for years accepted as final."[16]

WHY THIS DOCTOR QUESTIONS FLU VACCINATION

by Damien Downing, M.D.

The year of the vaccine showdown may have been 2009, the moment when enough of us started questioning all we're being told about vaccines. A survey published in the *British Medical Journal* reported that less than half of health-care workers in Hong Kong were willing to accept "pre-pandemic" flu vaccination.[18] And that was before a letter from the Health Protection Agency was sent to neurologists in the United Kingdom, warning them about increased cases of Guillain-Barré syndrome following the vaccination campaign. When nurses and doctors start questioning vaccination for themselves, patients should also be advised to make up their own minds. They seem to be doing so anyway. Another poll found that 51 percent thought taking the H1N1 vaccine carried a greater risk than not being vaccinated.[19] Yet, in both the U.S. and the U.K., this year's swine flu vaccine will be rolled out without adequate safety testing. What's going on? Two things: profits and power.

- Profits: Pharmaceutical companies love pandemics. They are a great way to sell practically useless drugs such as Tamiflu. A review by the Centre for Reviews and Dissemination at York University found that these drugs reduced the duration of flu symptoms by less than a day and recommended that giving them to healthy adults "is unlikely to be the most appropriate course of action."[20] But drug manufacturers clean up to the tune of $50 billion per year from influenza vaccines alone,[21] on a vaccine without proper safety testing and with efficacy totally unproven. A 2005 study was unable to "correlate increasing vaccination coverage after 1980 with declining mortality rates in any age group." Instead, they attributed the reduction in deaths to acquired "herd" immunity—nothing to do with vaccines.[22]

- Power: Governments love pandemics. Lots of sick people supports a system in which compulsory vaccination is imposed against our will, and where nutrients, which can provide cheap, safe, and effective treatments for many problems, are being outlawed on the basis of manipulated and flawed evidence.[23] The term *biopower* was first coined by French philosopher Michel Foucault to describe the use by governments of technologies to control populations—that is, to control our bodies. Vaccination is a good example of this; a technology that governments seek to impose on us, ostensibly to prevent a harm, such as death and damaged health.

Take autism as an example. What is the risk of developing autism if you get all or most of the long list of vaccinations for children? It is one in sixty-four in children ages five to nine, according to Professor Baron-Cohen, director of the Autism Research Centre, in Cambridge. Add in older kids still hobbled by autism spectrum disorders (ASD) and younger ones yet to be diagnosed, and you get approximately 100,000 autistic children in the U.K. Most swine flu vaccine contains thimerosal, a preservative that is nearly 50 percent mercury, and this is probably a major cause of autism. A proper risk analysis of flu vaccinations would identify the chance of autism as the greater likely cost, both human cost to the individual and financial to the state. Fair discussion of risk is prevented by management of the information flow.

The swine flu virus that caused the outbreak in 1977 "was probably an accidental release from a laboratory source."[24] During that outbreak, the U.S. launched a mass vaccination campaign, but this led to at least twenty-five deaths and 500 cases of Guillain-Barré syndrome; there were also thousands of injury claims. This time around, to protect their profits, the vaccine manufacturers clearly needed immunity from prosecution, which has now been granted to them.

The Real Solution—The conventional advice on how to protect yourself from swine flu is to stay away from other people, wear a mask, get vaccinated, take Tamiflu, and so on. But the real solution, the one you rarely hear about, is nutritional. There is plenty of evidence for nutritional intake making a difference to your risk of developing flu symptoms, to the development of complications, and to your time for recovery. Adults should consider taking the following (all doses are approximate and levels are safe):

- Vitamin D, 4,000 IU daily
- Vitamin A, 25,000 IU daily (unless you're pregnant or likely to become so)
- Vitamin C, 1,000 mg several times daily (at least)
- Zinc, 25 mg daily

The quantities may be scaled down for children, as described in Chapter 12.

See your doctor and talk this over. Read the small print, of course, and take other supplements if your body tells you it needs them. As for vaccination? That is, or at least should be, your decision.

(Dr. Downing, formerly editor of the *Journal of Nutritional and Environmental Medicine,* is currently president of the British Society for Allergy Environmental and Nutritional Medicine.)

[Commentary by Dr. Campbell: There has not been an honest discussion about thimerosal in vaccines; there has only been a fight. Even though the medical establishment (for lack of a better term) denies any association with the increased incidence of autism, they nevertheless removed thimerosal from several vaccines. It cannot be denied that mercury and other heavy metals are toxic to immature nervous systems and that they are cumulative. When we consider the fact that by one year of age, an infant is expected to receive eighteen shots (some with thimerosal), we have a toxic situation that must be honestly evaluated. Those shots could contain twenty-six antigens, a terrible jolt to an immature immune system, as well. There has to be honest discussion between the doctor (or other professional shot givers) and the parent. The problem is that parents are not prepared to question the "wisdom" of their doctor. I hope we can supply that motivation to better prepare. Then, if parents can't have such a discussion, I would hope they could find a doctor who welcomes an interchange of ideas that benefits both parties.]

Fortunately, this did not stop Dr. Klenner, who piloted megascorbate therapy for his patients during the 1948 polio epidemic. "For patients treated in the home," writes Dr. Klenner, "the dose schedule was 2,000 mg by needle every six hours, supplemented by 1,000 to 2,000 mg every two hours by mouth."[17] That is a total of 8,000 mg per day intramuscularly, plus, allowing for sleep, oral doses in the range of an additional 16,000–32,000 mg. This yields a total between 20,000 and 40,000 mg of vitamin C per day.

In the late 1970s, as a young father, and long before I had ever heard of Dr. Jungeblut, I was earnestly applying megadoses of ascorbate due to what I'd read by Drs. Stone and Klenner. Their papers, written standing solidly upon Dr. Jungeblut's shoulders, were the primary reason I was able to raise healthy children without Salk shots or Sabin sugar cubes. But my kids certainly took a lot of vitamin C. From seven decades past, Dr. Jungeblut has directly influenced the course of every orthomolecular practitioner and earned the thanks of every patient whose health, and life, has been saved by ascorbate therapy.

VACCINATIONS AND SCHOOLS

As a parent of a school-aged child, you will have to make decisions about the need versus the requirement of various vaccinations for your child. Unfortunately, in some states, it is as if the decision is made for you: the child must receive these vaccines prescribed by certain medical authoritative bodies. Also, states vary as to what kinds of exemptions are allowed—religious, medical, or moral. An informed parent should be allowed to decide, after conferring with the doctor, which vaccines are to be accepted or rejected. Doctors must be willing to discuss the pros and the cons.

Most schools, nationwide, require DtaP (diphtheria, tetanus, attenuated pertussis), IPV (inactivated poliovirus), MMR (mumps, measles, rubella)—all given in the form of a shot—upon entrance to school. If you have experienced the maze of possibly as many as nineteen shots (containing twenty-nine antigens) given to your infant by the age of one, you have been through the worst of it. We now are dealing with booster shots. Vaccines are made of components of bacteria or of live or attenuated viruses that will stimulate the immune system to form anti-bodies against them. The diphtheria and tetanus portions of the DtaP represent the oldest vaccines we have, even though they have been modified several times. It is hard to fault the "D" if we look at the pre-vaccination days, when so many children died of diphtheria. Tetanus vaccination has been the standard since its well-proven effect in World War One. There never seems to be a firm optimal interval recommended for boosters, but fortunately, tetanus is rare wherever good public health measures are in force. The pertussis (whooping cough) portion has been updated several times, but has never been shown to be a very good vaccine, in that vaccinated individuals often get the disease during an epidemic. Most infected people show little more than signs of a cold. It gets its name from the more serious phase: a patient starts to cough and can't stop until completely out of breath, then desperately draws in a breath through an inflamed larynx, causing a "whoop." Vomiting may follow as an attempt to reflexively clear the windpipe. The more serious aspects of the disease are mostly limited to infants and young children, so I see no need for pertussis protection for the school-age group. You may want to discuss with your health provider the possibility of switching to an adult version of the vaccine that leaves out the pertussis component.

The polio vaccine in use in this country is also given by shot. It has a good track record for safety and being free of side effects, and it remains effective for a long length of time. However, I (RC) think they are recommending booster shots too close together. But it probably isn't worth the hassle to protest—just go ahead and get it.

The only necessary use for a mumps vaccine is for the protection for boys who could develop the rare complication of orchitis (inflammation of the testicle), which leads very rarely to sterilization. When the MR vaccine was first developed, it was thought that it would provide lifelong protection, similar to having the natural disease. When tested later, it was found that protection dropped off to unacceptable levels after only eight years. A booster (after the first shot at 12–15 months) was then recommended for junior high students, administered as the newer MMR vaccine. However, I don't see why another booster is needed after only three to four years (the current recommendation).

Other Vaccines

Regarding the varicella (chicken pox) vaccination, I see no reason for it. I would like to get back to the old-fashioned situation in which nearly all susceptible people caught chicken pox in the spring, leaving very few adults vulnerable. I realize that it was a lot easier then for a mother to stay home with her mildly sick child, since she was generally not working. As far as the "shingles" shot for adults goes, it is not required. What we really all need is a general, nutritional boost of our immune systems, not a shot to prevent just one disease.

Considering the papilloma virus vaccine, at the onset I would advise answering with a firm "no." This virus is a cause of cervical cancer. It is very widespread, causing disease only when other mitigating conditions are present, such as multiple sex partners. In normal circumstances, natural immunity prevents disease. The vaccine has been revised after finding the lack of protection for strains not in the previous vaccine. But the safety record is poor: little is being said about its very serious side effects. The real travesty is in the campaign to vaccinate eleven-year-old girls before they are sexually active, a case of the "benevolent" pharmaceutical company looking out for our daughters and bypassing parental advice. Parents, you should have a choice, and the decision should be made following a discussion with your daughter. Beware: the next push to vaccinate preadolescent boys is already in progress.

IF NO VACCINES, WHAT THEN?

We look at the attempt to provide a vaccine for every infectious disease as side-stepping the real cause of infectious diseases. Our immune systems are in a mess due to poor nutrition, environmental toxin exposure, and other stressors. Correcting the causes of immunodeficiency will benefit every physiologic system. If a medicine cannot be

WHAT MAKES A GOOD PEDIATRICIAN

My (RC) hope is for every parent to find a good doctor for their children. Heaven forbid, but bad things happen—athletic injuries, medical emergencies involving trouble breathing, and lesser things that are not really "lesser," such as getting your doctor's help in navigating the regulatory hurdles that can enable you to reject an unwanted, unnecessary vaccination.

While applying what you learn in this book about orthomolecular medicine and realizing the individual differences in effective doses, a medical emergency could arise. Recently, I looked at Dr. Lendon Smith's book *Feed Your Kids Right*. He was a pediatrician who had a popular radio show and was among the first to employ orthomolecular medicine megadoses of vitamins, particularly vitamin C. At the same time, he hoped that standard medical care and orthomolecular medicine could work together. I am certain that if Dr. Smith were alive today, he would agree that antibiotic misuse and immunizations have gotten out of hand but that it would be unwise to abandon all professional care. He listed several bacterial infections that he felt should be treated with antibiotics, such as bacterial meningitis. Self-diagnosis is not needed. If a child is "sick"—having trouble breathing, experiencing a headache, weak, or barely responsive—every parent knows that immediate attention by a trained health professional is needed. An honest discussion about a treatment plan should follow. It will take time for you to discover your child's individual need for megadoses of vitamin C that will prevent, favorably modify, or cure various illnesses. If you find a "listening" doctor for your child, hang on to him or her.

A children's doctor should be, above all, supportive—a partner in childrearing, a wise detector of the potential for physical problems, and a guide to the safest, most efficient ways to head them off. Periodic complete physical examinations, accompanied by questions both asked and answered, are essential. There will come a time when an athletic physical examination is required. This can be just a cursory, regulation-satisfying exam or an opportunity for a question-and-answer session, requiring a solid doctor–patient relationship to deal with potential injuries. Plus, insurance coverage demands it. A doctor can also help steer you down the regulatory path of vaccination requirements. And while one never wants to experience a medical emergency, if something should occur, it is infinitely better to deal with a familiar doctor.

Following orthomolecular principles should help you "keep the doctor away" better than the daily apple (though that might be continued as well). But there will be times when one is needed. A doctor who dismisses any consideration of preventive health measures through nutrition, including supplements, does not fit the bill. He or she must carefully evaluate the need for antibiotics, vaccinations, or medicines on a case-by-case basis and demonstrate a willingness to work *with* the parent. This type of doctor is less plentiful in sparsely populated areas because, unfortunately, insurance does not reimburse for this kind of service.

The best method of finding the doctor you need is through referral from your friends. If your present arrangement is not working, look elsewhere, but don't entirely cut yourself off from care.

found for an illness, the industry strives to come up with a vaccine. The truth concerning the need for and the effectiveness of various vaccines requires open discussion, and a consent form pressed upon a parent at the moment of injection will not suffice.

One obvious question is: "What do you do if you are not vaccinating your children and they actually became ill from a disease?" Healthy eating and a strong immune system is key, but parents may want to set up a plan of action other than prevention. This is necessary because many pediatricians believe parents are uneducated if they choose not to vaccinate. So, if one of your children becomes ill, your pediatrician may not be on your side. It might be more of an "I told you so" mentality.

Now, the worst-case scenario is that a child is so sick as to perhaps require hospitalization. If it gets this bad, parents simply cannot leave the final decision to the doctors, and that's assuming you have doctors that will listen at all. Parents must know the facts about orthomolecular therapy, particularly vitamin C megadoses (see Part Four of this book). Also, the next chapter offers tips on how to boost immune function naturally.

SUMMARY

There has been a mad rush to eliminate disease by developing antibiotics for bacterial disease and vaccines for viral and bacterial diseases. It seems that viruses and bacteria, having been on Earth far longer than we humans, have learned more survival tricks. Mutating bacteria have manufacturers of antibiotics and bacterial vaccines hustling to develop effective products. The same can be said for the virus vaccines. In spite of decades of warnings to those prescribing antibiotic treatment to use them cautiously and appropriately, the advice goes mainly unheeded. Long before a vaccine can be proven effective, the organism that is being fought changes its stripes, necessitating a new, untested vaccine. Our only true defense lies in what should be our primary defense: do everything we can to bolster our immune systems.

CHAPTER 4

How to Boost Your Child's Immune System Without Booster Shots

"It is time to lay to rest the notion that germs jump into people and cause diseases."
—Emanuel Cheraskin, M.D., D.M.D.

So there I (AWS) was in Africa, in a castle dungeon and looking up at a ceiling entirely covered with bats. My feet were Crocodile Hunter–deep in "bat poo" (guano), which had no discernable odor. It must have been a very different smell indeed back in the 1500s, when hundreds of slaves were held in this miserable stone cellar and others like it. Ventilation was by a single small barred window way up high. This particular fortress at Elmina in Ghana, West Africa, was once among the world's largest collecting and holding stations for slaves before they were shipped overseas. For those imprisoned here then, there was no running water, no toilets, and no hope. Today, it is promoted as a tourist destination. Do not let the shining white exterior fool you: Elmina Castle is truly an awful place on the inside, particularly underneath in those dungeons. The slaving business went on for nearly 400 years—organized oppression on a large commercial scale.

But on this day in 1974, down in the dungeon, lit by a single electric bulb, I saw nothing except bats. Thousands of them. Bats navigate by echolocation, meaning the stealthy little creatures have on-board sonar. By sending out high-pitched pulses and listening to their return, bats can fly around dungeons in the dark without ever hitting the walls or each other, or, incidentally, without ever getting in your hair.

Bats also find their food this way. Many bats like to eat moths. There are moth species that not only can hear the bat's sonar, but when they do hear it will automatically fold up their wings and fall several meters straight down. By the time the bat gets to where the moth is, it is where the moth was. The moth does something of an aikido (avoidance) move: it outmaneuvers its assailant.

The analogous aikido move in immunology is to strengthen an individual's immune system. It is futile to focus on the preemptive killing of every germ, every time, everywhere. It cannot be done. But rather than live inside a bubble, scramble for the latest antibiotic, or panic if your vaccination card is incomplete, why not concentrate on the many ways you can fortify your child's immune system? Most children could use a good health tune-up.

SWIMMING DUCKS OR SITTING DUCKS?

Ducks swim in water but do not get wet. This is because they have oiled their feathers to form a natural barrier that is impervious to moisture. We can do something similar with our immune systems.

We live in a world full of germs. Most of them are harmless and many are actually beneficial. Cows, by the way, cannot really eat grass, but the digestive bacteria in the cow's rumen can. Ultimately, they are to thank for the milk. Helpful bacteria in your digestive tract make you healthy too. Some bacteria actually make vitamins for you—notably B_6, B_{12}, and K—and some help break down your food and help process wastes.

Yes, some bacteria are nasty. But if the body is healthy, bacteria, pathogenic or not, are largely irrelevant. Consider this: horses' guts are full of tetanus bacteria, yet horses do not get tetanus via the gut. Or this: London sewer rats (which are always a tad hungry) live in an environment surrounded by filth and germs, but they are very hardy. On the other hand, white laboratory rats are kept nice and clean and are lovingly overfed; they die at the drop of a hat.

Our medicalized world is full to the brim with antibiotic over-prescription, and a resultant rise in the number of drug-resistant bacteria. We may soon see a dramatic increase in drug-resistant super-bacteria as antibiotics continue to be overused in humans and animals. The importance of utilizing harmless natural modalities to boost the immune system with which nature endowed us is, therefore, more important than ever.

TEN WAYS TO WRECK A CHILD'S IMMUNE SYSTEM

First, we'll look at what not to do. There are sure-fire ways to damage the effectiveness of the immune system. If you see any of your habits on this list, consider changing your ways for the health of your family.

1. Smoke near them.

2. Demonstrate how you can drink liberal quantities of alcohol, and let your kids drink plenty of soda pop until they are old enough for beer and booze.

3. Eat all the junk foods advertised on TV, especially lots of meat and sugar, and foods with chemical colors, flavors, and preservatives.

4. Never exercise.

5. Worry constantly. Just turn on TV news programs to help you accomplish this.

6. Take powerful antibiotics preventively.

7. Count on your daily diet for all the vitamins and minerals that your body really needs.

8. Make excuses to not read *How to Live Longer and Feel Better* by Linus Pauling.

9. Stay up late, and let the kids do so as well.

10. Regularly use a wide variety of over-the-counter drugs.

IMMUNE SYSTEM BOOSTERS

A healthy immune system is built every day by your lifestyle choices, especially your nutritional choices.

Immune Booster #1: Vitamin C

Take lots of vitamin C to help defend yourself against viruses and bacteria. For children, age-appropriate forms include vitamin C powder in juice (1,000 mg is a quarter-teaspoonful) or a couple of citrus-flavored 500-mg chewtabs (very tasty).

Immune Booster #2: Sleep

Conquer chronic tiredness. Get to bed earlier. Set the video recorder and watch that TV show tomorrow. You can get a more satisfying night's sleep by darkening your room: the darker your sleeping environment, the more melatonin (the sleep hormone) you make. Having a regular sleep pattern is very helpful. Homework and recreation times may need adjustment. Deep sleep is associated with the normal release of growth hormone in children.

Immune Booster #3: Research Natural Therapies

Strengthen your resolve reading scientific studies on the antitoxic, antibiotic, and antiviral properties of megadoses of vitamin C. We discuss other vitamins in Chapter 13.

Immune Booster #4: Multivitamin

Take a good multivitamin every day. Emanuel Cheraskin, M.D., D.M.D., writes that placebo-controlled research has shown people who take supplements have "higher numbers of certain T-cell subsets and natural killer cells, increased interleukin-2 production, and higher antibody response and natural killer cell activity." The result? Vitamin-takers were sick only half as many days per year as those who did not take supplements. Yet most Americans do not meet even the minimum standards for dietary adequacy.[1]

ORTHOMOLECULAR MEDICINE PIONEER: EMANUEL CHERASKIN, M.D., D.M.D.

Emanuel Cheraskin (1916–2001), born in Philadelphia, received his M.D. from the University of Cincinnati College of Medicine. He was awarded his D.M.D in the first graduating class of the University of Alabama School of Dentistry, where he would stay for several decades as chairman of the Department of Oral Medicine. Dr. Cheraskin was among the first to recognize and demonstrate that oral health indicates total body health. He wrote over 700 scientific articles and authored or co-authored seventeen textbooks, plus eight more books for the public, including the bestseller *Psychodietetics: Food as the Key to Emotional Health.* His last two books, *Vitamin C: Who Needs It?* and *Human Health and Homeostasis* were published when he was past eighty years old.

"Health is the fastest growing failing business in Western civilization," Dr. Cheraskin once stated. "Why is it so many of us are forty going on seventy, and so few seventy going on forty?" The answer, he said, was our neglect of the paramount value of nutrition, an educational deficiency that Dr. Cheraskin devoted a lifetime to eradicating.[2]

Immune Booster #5: Vitamin E

Take supplemental vitamin E. Placebo-controlled, double-blind trials have shown that 800 IU of vitamin E per day can improve immune responsiveness and immunocompetence. Plus, the response was seen in only thirty days.[3] A dose of 400 IU is probably enough for children up to adolescent age. For the little ones, open up the ends of a capsule and squeeze the contents into a bit of their favorite fruit juice. Be sure the preparation is natural or d-alpha tocopherol, which is much more effective than the synthetic dl-alpha tocopherol. Better yet, if it's not too expensive, look for natural mixed tocopherols at your health food store.

Immune Booster #6: Carotenes

Drink lots of vegetable juices, and here are some reasons why. Carotenes, the pigments that give fruits and vegetables orange colors, have been specifically shown in high doses to strengthen the immune system by helping the body to build more helper T cells. The amount used in one well-controlled study was 180 mg of beta-carotene per day. This is, theoretically at least, the equivalent of 300,000 IU of vitamin A per day (6 mg of beta-carotene can be converted into 10,000 IU of vitamin A in the body). That amount, consumed as the oil or retinol form of vitamin A, would likely be toxic, but as carotene it is not. There is indeed a big difference between forms. Also, the study produced positive results in a mere two weeks.[4] Even people with the weakest of immune systems, such as AIDS patients, can benefit from huge carotene dosages.[5]

Some have claimed that excess carotene consumption is dangerous. Excess carotene causes the skin to turn slightly orange (hypercarotenosis), once succinctly described as resembling an artificial suntan. Hypercarotenemia refers to elevated blood levels of carotene. Both hypercarotenosis and hypercarotenemia are harmless. Excess intake of carotene does not cause hypervitaminosis A.[6]

Immune Booster #7: Stop Smoking

What is the greatest preventable danger to the greatest number of people? The answer is, smoking. In the U.S. alone, tobacco kills fifty-one people an hour. Of course, the tobacco industry spends over $11 million every day on advertising to encourage this. Don't fall for it: research suggests that less smoking around children means fewer ear infections.[7]

A naturally strong immune system effectively resists disease. If it didn't, we would be extinct. Take the steps above to heart and we have a special advantage in addition to our opposable thumbs: we can substantially strengthen our immune systems, right now, and without prescription.

FIRST-HAND ACCOUNTS
OF SECOND-HAND SMOKE

Between the ages of six and nine months, "Jimmy" must have been to see me (RC) at least six times for middle ear infection—that is, the *beginning* of a middle ear infection. Jimmy always exhibited all the signs of a nasal allergy. His mother was an intelligent woman and, in general, a very good mom, but her clothes always reeked of tobacco smoke. She was a nicotine addict. I was careful in my attempts to help Jimmy get free of this allergen, for I knew that no matter what, his mother would think that I was saying she was a lousy mother. With each visit, my frustration increased until, at the last visit, she bundled up Jimmy and stormed out of the office. I blew it, right? A few months later, I and many other townspeople observed her running every morning to work, free of the "evil weed." Some told me that Jimmy was doing well too. It was a very satisfactory result.

The second case had an identical medical history but, unlike the first case, this young mother believed what I told her. She was a bright Native American mother who worked in an office in the Tribal Complex. I had visited some of those offices prior to the days of smoking bans and visibility was literally reduced to the length of the room. Coffee and smoke breaks, mandated by law, took place several times a day *in situ*. After the first examination of her infant for a suspected ear infection, she started the program we worked out. I explained that the addiction had a grip on her and that it would require a lot of fortitude on her part to kick it. I prescribed vitamins C and B-complex and advised her to begin an exercise program in good air. She immediately caught the concept of habits that were reinforcing one another—smoking, coffee, sweet rolls, chit-chat. Her solution was to go outside on her coffee breaks, leave the old habits behind, and run around the complex building. She started slow with the exercise program, but then steadily increased the distance and intensity. She kicked the habit(s), her little girl thrived, and I was one happy doctor.

In retrospect, years later, in spite of many opportunities to help adults stop smoking, my only successes were if there were circumstances similar to these two cases. A mother will make huge sacrifices if her child's health requires them, but she may not do it just for her own sake. Getting free of nicotine addiction is tough, but do it for your kids and yourself. I have found that taking a vitamin B preparation (B-50) once a day is a great aid during the withdrawal period. A strong incentive to quit coupled with a change in associated bad habits, plus the B vitamins, are going to work better than anti-smoking medicines or a different form of nicotine.

SCARED OF DISEASE?

Nursing and medical students have a fairly high rate of hypochondria. This is due to their necessarily obsessive study of pathology, a topic that is enough to make anyone feel a little sickened. The public too, from time to time, is subjected to media-driven obsession with loathsome diseases. This is nothing new. Leprosy, a relatively non-contagious disease, has been widely feared since Biblical times. The pox, the plague, polio, and pertussis have all had their day in the news, and not without reason. But sometimes we do well to step back a bit and look at the big picture.

What really used to scare me (AWS) was tuberculosis (TB). I was an avid reader and I'd read too many graphic accounts of helpless, ashen-faced TB patients spitting up ghastly red blood as they slowly wasted away from "consumption." In fact, my Public Health Explorer Post met in an old sanitarium wing of a former TB hospital. There we learned how to propagate (harmless) bacteria, and to loop, stain, and identify them.

At age eighteen, while waiting for a train at London's Euston Station, I was unavoidably involved in a conversation with a drunken derelict in search of an easy 50 pence. As he coughed virtually in my face, he told me he had recently gotten out of prison. He sought to prove his honesty by producing tattered but nonetheless official green

Her Majesty's Prison discharge papers. I happened to read, as he continued coughing, that he also had been diagnosed with tuberculosis. I gave him the 50p to get rid of him and breathe clean air again. For a long time afterward, I worried that I'd get TB.

Oddly enough, when I first taught college, the only job I could get was in penitentiaries. My "captive audience" also coughed a great deal. Back then, one in eight prisoners tested positive for TB (the current figure is better than one in four). I spent many hours in badly ventilated rooms with a lot of very unhealthy men and women. As a condition of employment, prison faculty had to have TB tests. Mine remained negative.

Tuberculosis is bacterial, while polio is viral and, to many, all the more dreadful. As my unvaccinated kids grew up, confrontational adults would often ask, "What would you do if your children got polio?" The answer is, follow the instructions of Drs. Frederick R. Klenner and Robert F. Cathcart on how to cure serious viral illnesses with large doses of vitamin C. But the royal road is to see that your children don't get sick in the first place. You keep people healthy by feeding them right, which means a plant-based, vitamin-supplemented diet. Few questioners' patience would last long enough for me to say all that. They would come back with, "But you can't prevent polio; it's a virus!" Substitute "whooping cough" or any of the public's favorite dreaded diseases, and you have another batch of prefabricated, fear-based, panic-driven debates. And yet they all have a common solution: prevent with diet; cure with vitamin C.

People have the idea that "germs," either bacteria or viruses, are the primary cause of disease. This is not true. The scare for many is swine flu, Ebola virus, West Nile fever, or any of a number of biological bogeymen trumpeted by the news media. It is a shame that the same news media has not devoted a single minute to how to cure bacterial and viral illnesses with vitamin C megadoses. (For more on vitamin therapy, see Part Four of this book.)

SUMMARY

It is impossible to be free of disease by thinking that we can take care of disease-producing agents one at a time with an antibiotic or a vaccine. If we boost every function of the immune system, we not only go a long way toward the prevention of infectious diseases but we will also enhance its capabilities in cancer and heart disease prevention. The latter conditions take years to develop—we need to start our children on what works as soon as we learn it.

We don't want our little ones living in filth, but we are learning that some exposure to "germs" early in life can get the immune system in gear and actually be helpful. So, we need not strive for a sterile environment. Bacteria and humans are evolving together. If the truth be known, without help for our immune systems, the bacteria will win. We know the good effect of antioxidants, including those found in fresh, ripe, naturally-brightly-colored fruits and vegetables. We need not succumb to the fear produced by pharmaceutical advertising, if we counter it with truthful knowledge and practices.

PART TWO

STAYING HEALTHY WITH DIET AND DETOXIFICATION

CHAPTER 5

WHAT IS THE HEALTHIEST
DIET FOR YOUR CHILD?

*"He who lives by rule and wholesome diet
is a physician to himself."*
—FROM CONCISE DIRECTIONS ON THE NATURE OF OUR
COMMON FOOD SO FAR AS IT TENDS TO PROMOTE OR
INJURE HEALTH (LONDON: SWORDS OF LONDON, 1790)

Pediatricians used to be mailed a *Pediatric Nutrition Handbook* every few years. I (RC) was revisiting my old 1979 book and what a cruel joke it was! The description of vitamins and the recommended doses was appalling. In the back, under "Additional Reading," were titles such as "Nutrition Misinformation and Food Faddism" and "Food Cultism and Nutrition Quackery." And guess who the "quacks" were? Linus Pauling, Abram Hoffer, and Benjamin Feingold. Addressing Dr. Feingold's hypothesis that additives create bad behavior in children, the *Pediatric Nutrition Handbook* states that "most physicians prefer to recommend therapies of unambiguous efficacy. The Feingold diet has not attained that status."

I beg to differ. I had a case that dramatized the Feingold theory. I don't remember the date but it must have been shortly before 1979. The parents knew of my interest in allergies and brought their son to me. He had twice been "saved" by administering adrenaline in an emergency room for what they described as classic angioneurotic edema (swelling beneath the skin). Fortunately, they believed what I said about searching for the offending allergenic substance: list absolutely *every* ingredient in everything eaten or drunk preceding the event by only a short time. On the third E.R. visit, we hit the jack-pot—the culprit was Red Dye #2, present in a breakfast cereal (I believe it was Fruit Loops). Eliminating this substance from their son's diet meant no more trips to the E.R.

Perhaps it is time to stop taking nutrition advice from the same professionals who brought you hospital food. Medical students are taught very little about nutrition in medical school, and it shows. A healthy diet can have a profound impact on your children's development and growth, helping them to stay well and avoid illness.

WHY YOU ARE SICK IF YOU WANT TO EAT RIGHT

First of all, we are not making this up. "Healthy Food Obsession Sparks Rise in New Eating Disorder: Fixation with Healthy Eating Can Be Sign of Serious Psychological Disorder" was an actual headline from *The Observer*, the United Kingdom's oldest Sunday newspaper, found-ed in 1791. Concern about eating right now has an official disease name: orthorexia nervosa.[1] Symptoms evidently include "refusing to touch sugar, salt, caffeine, alcohol, wheat, gluten, yeast, soya, corn and dairy foods, [and] any foods that have come into contact with pesti-cides, herbicides or contain artificial additives." Also, "sufferers tend to be aged over 30, middle-class and well-educated" and "solely con-cerned with the quality of the food they put in their bodies."[2]

Comic strip artist Morrie Brickman once quipped, "I don't know if the world is full of smart men bluffing or imbeciles who mean it." Orthorexia nervosa is not a prank, but is should be seen for the non-sense it is. A "fixation with healthy eating" is, well, healthy. After all, if you are not a health nut, then just what kind of a nut are you?

Following are our suggestions for healthy eating, for you and your children.

DR. CAMPBELL'S VIEW ON DIET

Diet is a word that we hear constantly in the media—the same media that informs us of medical "breakthroughs" in the treatment of most every chronic disorder. From this persistence, many then equate "diet" with a medicine, and there seems to be a separate diet for weight loss, cardiovascular disease, energy enhancement, rheumatoid arthritis, and other chronic diseases. But diet should be thought of more often as the basis for disease prevention and not just something to get one out of a health problem. On top of an ideal preventive diet, add vitamin supplements and you are on your way to good health.

America's biggest health problem is obesity and the spin-off diseases associated with it. Just as the search for a cure for cancer is not a realistic goal, so it is with medicine or surgery to "cure" obesity. The diets with doctor's names attached—Atkins, Ornish, and Sears—each have great attributes that can apply to many aspects of health, but they have been pitted against each other in the quest to lose weight.

For a broader approach to a good prevention diet, we have looked at the general diet of regions where the older population is healthier than ours. Personally, I think I would do very well on a Mediterranean diet if I could consider the whole program and not just the olive oil and red wine. The Japanese and Israeli traditional diets have done very well for their peoples. Unfortunately, Western food culture is creeping in, along with stress, cigarettes, and other pollutants. What we have to do is look at all these diets in which longevity is enhanced and separate the "good" nutritional factors from the "bad." We live here, after all, and we can concoct our own special diet by this type of analysis.

In defining an ideal "healthiest" diet, first remove the "bad" factors. Processed foods, so prevalent in the American diet, have had their content of vitamins and minerals altered and are not processed properly in our bodies. Fats are often changed to the point where our bodies don't recognize them as nutrients. Sugar should be minimized: we get sufficient fruit sugar (fructose) from fruit and need to consider soda, with its unnaturally huge high-fructose corn syrup content, a rare (if at all) treat. Our meat intake should be cut way back. There are a myriad of chemicals added to processed foods, designed to make the foods more salable, but making them less like foods. Our bodies are not equipped to metabolize them, so be sure to avoid "foods" that are anything but natural.

The base of a healthy diet is food we describe with a variety of adjectives: whole, natural (unadulterated), organic, or fresh—the other side of what we just described. If one can find it available and affordable, "organic," as it pertains to produce, meat, eggs, and dairy foods, encompasses the other descriptive words. Organic produce, grown in soil that follows the standards of certified organic farming, will have a higher level of trace minerals and phyto-antioxidants (potent and plant-based). The produce has a better chance of being harvested at the optimal time to aid flavor and freshness, and maximize nutrient content,. And, of course, it is free or close to free of pesticides. If you can talk to a local producer, you might find one who is 80 percent eligible for organic certification but can't qualify because of a limiting (nonsignificant) regulation.

Organic meat comes from grass-fed and not feedlot-fattened animals. The difference is in the fatty acid content of the animal's fat: omega-3s in the grass fed, omega-6s in the grain fed. This equates to less promotion of inflammation. Organic milk comes from cows given organic feed that also have not been given injections of artificial bovine growth hormone (BGH). BGH is used to increase milk production beyond the time it would naturally decline. Unfortunately, it greatly increases the incidence of mastitis and the need to treat the sick animal with antibiotics. Both the hormone and antibiotics can enter into commercial milk. Other countries have banned this practice, but the U.S. Department of Agriculture won't even allow labeling milk that comes from treated cows.

Compare the yolks of eggs from organically raised chickens versus "cooped-up" chickens raised on commercial egg farms. The difference in the depth of color of the yolks depicts the difference in phyto-antioxidant levels. There are no antibiotics or pesticides in organically raised chickens or their eggs. Labeling a product "organic" or "natural" promotes sales, so be sure to make certain the product is what it claims to be on the label.

Making the Switch to a Healthier Diet

It is a major undertaking to switch from a typical diet, heavily weighted in processed food and drink, to a whole-foods diet. First of all, be completely convinced that it is the right thing to do and that it has to be done, then the whole family can inspire one another. If you have friends who eat healthy, let them help.

A good place to start is with breakfast. Try a multi-grained hot cereal to replace the dry cereal in a box. This change requires a bit more preparation time and a show of love and concern as you chip away at old habits and acquire new ones. The new cereal has a different (probably less sugary) flavor and texture, but it has a good chance of actually tasting better. You might need to make a more gradual transition by starting with as natural a dry cereal as you can find, one free of sugar, chemicals, and artificial coloring. Breakfast should be a "stick-to-the-ribs" meal: eggs, yogurt, and even a "little" meat will supply the protein and fat that makes the meal more sustaining. Fruit, as long as it is taken with these foods, also goes well.

Successfully introducing strange new foods requires creativity. Vegetables may have been rejected in the past due to the practice of overcooking, rendering them unattractive, tasteless, and with fiber content providing the only speck of nutritional value. Learn to barely cook (steam) them. Salads are a wonderful way to enjoy raw vegetables. Some leftover cooked vegetables can be added, and several fruits blend nicely with greens. Markets often carry convenient packages of organic salad greens. A good salad dressing (read the label to make sure it is junk free) applied in small amounts is not prohibitive. When new habits are better established, think of creative ways of presenting more raw vegetables, such as "as is" or run through a juicer. The opportunities for more fruit intake are easier—as snack material, with regular meals, or blended with yogurt as a "smoothie." When shopping for vegetables and fruits, a simple rule applies: deep, rich colors are correlated with a good content of phyto-antioxidants.

If availability or cost discourage you from purchasing organic foods, settle for next best. Look for produce that is fresh and harvested when ripe (even vegetables picked when they are "nature ready"). You can eliminate pesticide residues by peeling vegetables and fruits, and reduce residues by thoroughly washing leafy greens and other vegetables with a dilute soap solution (followed by rinsing, of course). I know that in my area, when home gardens are dormant in winter, there is a paucity of fresh produce in our (otherwise) "super" markets: broccoli, root vegetables, a short period of availability of winter squash, and organic "greens." If this is the case, frozen vegetables and fruits might be the only viable option. At least they have been processed only after they achieve ripeness, with far less heat than is used in canning or bottling.

Strive to take meat out of its status as the star of the meal; reduce it to "best supporting actor" in a subordinate capacity. Organic meat is more costly, but the cost can easily be offset—just eat less of it. Whole-grain pasta should replace nutrient-poor regular pasta (expect a taste treat). The same goes for whole-grain breads and rice; they are both very tasty and infinitely better for you.

When we attempt to get in shape, we don't start out by running a marathon, but we do have to *start*. If your diet patterns need a complete turnabout, begin the gradual learning process. There is more to eating than taking in nutrients. Meals are a great time to have family conversation around the table: conversation slows the mechanical process of eating, which may induce weight loss by helping you reflect more on what you are eating as opposed to simply bolting down food without enjoyment. It is a good time for finding out what is going on in your children's lives.

DR. SAUL'S VIEW: A PLANT-BASED DIET, BUT NOT NECESSARILY VEGETARIAN

The health benefits of a plant-based diet impress even the U.S. Food and Drug Administration. At their website, they quote registered dietitian Johanna Dwyer, of Tufts University Medical School and the New England Medical Center Hospital in Boston, who states the following plant-food benefits: "Data are strong that vegetarians are at lesser risk for obesity, atonic [reduced muscle tone] constipation, lung cancer, and alcoholism. Evidence is good that risks for hypertension, coronary artery disease, type II diabetes, and gallstones are lower."[3]

Although the word *vegetarian* is often a source of contention, the qualifier *near* should be the focal point for discussion. The recent Cornell University China studies clearly support near-vegetarianism (up to 20 percent animal-based foods), which is our preferred long-term dietary maintenance plan. Cornell University's extensive nutrition studies have shown that people eating little or no animal protein are less likely to get either cancer or heart disease. "Disease patterns in much of rural China tend to reflect those prior to the industrial revolution in the U.S., when cancers and cardiovascular diseases were much less prevalent."[4]

Decades earlier, researchers such as Francis Pottenger, M.D., and Dr. Weston Price had repeatedly shown that "primitive" peoples or laboratory animals eating a natural (but not vegetarian) diet did not have serious diseases.

Raw Foods

I generally recommend that everyone endeavor to follow the spirit of Dr. Pottenger's message: less cooked food, more raw food. If and when food is cooked, make sure it is as unprocessed as possible. Minimal cooking and minimal processing means maximum vitamin and nutrient content.

Dr. Pottenger's emphasis was on the nutritional value of raw foods, and he got it right. He knew that carnivorous animals, normally, would never be in a position to hunt a cooked meal. His studies were primarily on cats, and most felines are carnivores. But even carnivores are not strictly carnivorous: lions and similar predators gobble up the predigested vegetable material from an herbivorous prey animal's digestive organs in preference to any other part of the kill. I caught my cat up on the kitchen counter the other day. She was eating carrot pulp left over from the morning's juicing. Years ago, I had a cat that would stand up on her hind legs and beg for cooked green beans. But this was in addition to an appropriately meaty kitty diet, including the cat's quite raw "catch of the day" mouse or mole from the garden.

For humans, if a vegetable, fruit, or dairy food can be eaten uncooked, then it should be. It is obvious to anyone who has opened a can of vegetables or eaten a stewed prune that there is more fiber, and taste, in raw fruits and vegetables. Raw milk, from scrupulously clean dairies, is itself clean. When I was a dairy farmer, I fed my own young kids raw milk right from the "tap": from udder to milk tank

to child. This was over thirty years ago. Today, it is increasingly difficult to locate a farmer or dairy that can supply raw milk without
running afoul of legal restrictions. Look for "Certified Raw Milk" at
health food stores.

As for raw meat, well, no thank you. The Natural Hygienists have
what is at heart the same message: eat fresh and raw. I admire and
seek to emulate such knowledge to the maximum practical extent, but
I do not apologize for having a stove. A whole-food, good food diet
including legumes (peas, beans, lentils), grains, and potatoes clearly
needs some cooking. But there is definitely no need to make one's
home on the range.

Native Diets

You cannot go far wrong eating along the dietary lines of the healthy,
traditional cultures that Dr. Price visited and described. Dr. Price
found that isolated, robust Swiss communities ate cheese and raw
milk daily, plus a lot of whole-grain bread, but they ate meat only
once a week. The basic foods of the islanders of the Outer Hebrides,
Dr. Price wrote, "are fish and oat products with a little barley. Oat
grain . . . provides the porridge and oat cakes, which in many homes
are eaten in some form regularly with every meal."[5] Even traditional Eskimos, often held up as the ultimate example of human carnivores, also eat nuts along with "kelp stored for winter use, berries
including cranberries, which are preserved by freezing, blossoms of
flowers preserved in seal oil, [and] sorrel grass preserved in seal oil."[6]

When I personally visited rural Africa (some thirty-five years after
Dr. Price), I saw surprisingly healthy people. This was a slight shock
to my Western expectations. I also saw what most people were eating: garden vegetables and whole grains. In every village, there seemed
to be a big drum of boiling water containing steamed corn on the
cob. Along the roadside, people sometimes sold a delicacy that closely resembled a dried, whole woodchuck. I passed on that, but I also
found bananas for sale everywhere. They were small but right off the
tree and sweet as gumdrops. As in China, rural Africans appear to
eat what their poverty brings them, and that is mostly what they can

catch and what they can grow. Practically speaking, subsistence agriculture is a more sure thing economically than subsistence hunting is. It supports more people, and it is healthier.

In short, most "vegetarians" are not, and most "carnivores" are not. The optimum human diet is not to be found at either extreme. The issue is natural food more than where it comes from. Unprocessed foods, whether of animal or plant origin, are the healthiest. This is the enduring message of Drs. Price and Pottenger.

That "V" word, vegetarian, stops many a free exchange of ideas. Let's make it perfectly clear: this is about good, sensible moderation, not polarizing absolutes. It is more important to eat whole, high-fiber, low-sugar natural foods. Cooking, minimize. Meat, minimize. That does not mean "no" or none!

MEAT: LOTS, SOME, OR NONE?

Americans consume about three times as much protein as they need. Worldwide, 30 g of protein daily is usually considered adequate. The U.S. Recommended Dietary Allowance (RDA) of protein is much more generous than that, about 60 g daily for a man and about 50 g daily for a woman. However, we generally eat more than 100 g of protein daily, mostly from meat. Chronic protein excess can overload and irreversibly damage the kidneys by middle age.[7]

We eat too much protein. We eat too much fat as well. We need to cut down on both and eat more vegetables, beans, nuts, and fruits. The muscles of dead animals are simply not necessary for protein if you eat some dairy, some fish, and lots of legumes and fresh nuts. Near-vegetarianism makes sense on all levels. When in doubt, eat like other primates do. Chimps, gorillas, and orangutans are very strong, very smart, and mostly—but not entirely—vegetarian. By moving toward a vegetarian diet, you automatically reduce your excessive intake of protein, fat, and sugar. It is just that simple; there is no diet plan to buy. Dairy products, eggs, and fish must remain occasional options for most of us, and growing children generally do well as lacto-ovo-vegetarians.

Avoiding all animal products makes one a vegan. I (AWS) am most certainly not a vegan, and I do not universally advocate it. I have many good friends who utterly and totally reject animal products, and I admire them for this. I also observe that their conviction is, at times, more admirable than their health is. Ethical issues aside, veganism truly is an excellent transition diet. As limited-term treatment for overweight, constipated, drug-soaked people, veganism cannot be beat. I think a few months without animal products is worth a therapeutic trial for most illnesses. But long term, for most people, I think some animal foods are necessary as the decades pass.

The majority of vegetarians are actually near-vegetarians, eating some animal products, such as milk products. I am something of a cheese and yogurt fan (as a former dairyman, what do you expect?). I also use eggs now and then for cooking, but I am not much of a milk drinker. You will also need to discover your own balance among these options.

Albert Einstein wrote, "Nothing will benefit human health and increase the chances for survival of life on Earth as much as the evolution to a vegetarian diet." Evolution, a key word, means gradual change with time. Vegetarianism is a process, not an absolute.

Let's not let semantics be a stumbling block. Since "meatless" is taken to mean "meat free," may we suggest instead "less meat"? That most certainly does not mean "zero animal products." And when considering the moral arguments on the dialectics of dietetics, we are humbled when we recall that Mahatma Gandhi ate goat's milk and cheese, and Jesus ate fish. I cannot even be described as a lacto-ovo-vegetarian (dairy and eggs), for I also eat seafood, because fish and their oceanic mates are valuable nutrition sources. After millennia of changes to human civilization, the world's number one animal protein source is still seafood. By the time we come up with a definition of "fishatarian," we are very close to the natural animal-products percentages that Dr. Price found again and again in his travels among "primitive" (a.k.a. healthy) cultures.

More Reasons to Eat Less Meat

When considering meat consumption, I (AWS) suggest keeping in mind the following:

WORTH THE READ:
UPTON SINCLAIR'S *THE JUNGLE*

Upton Sinclair's *The Jungle* has absolutely nothing to do with either rain forests or the tropics. Rather, it is an exposé of the utter brutality of American meatpacking and meat processing industries. This famous 1906 novel has been widely acknowledged as responsible for bringing about the first U.S. Food and Drug Act, much in the same way that Harriet Beecher Stowe's novel *Uncle Tom's Cabin* helped raise a public uproar against slavery half a century earlier. Sinclair's intent was to show the harsh living conditions of America's working class and the corruption of the meatpacking industry, but the public's reaction was to the food not the workers. "I aimed at the public's heart, and by accident I hit it in the stomach," Sinclair later said.

Time has not diminished the book's punch. In this classic tale of industrial and agricultural misery, it is hard to tell who suffers more, the grimly impoverished human characters or the nameless animals that are cruelly slaughtered for ham, leather, and lard. It's a literary guided tour of a slaughterhouse, where you are virtually herded, right along with the workers and the cattle, through the muck of Chicago's stockyards to witness diseased animals being killed and ground into meat for sale.

This absolutely merciless book illustrates one of the major reasons people eat so many take-out burgers and packaged foods: to avoid confronting the realities of where our food comes from. Who wants this close a look at kill floors, blood, and rendering vats? But if you find *The Jungle* abhorrent, you are normal. A farmer friend of mine once said that what is truly disgusting are the tidy, plastic-wrapped packages of meat neatly displayed in supermarket coolers, for those are impossibly far from what the animal looked like when it was born, raised, killed, flayed and dismembered.

Not all packing plants are bad. Interestingly, Oprah Winfrey took some followers, including Michael Pollan, author of *The Omnivore's Dilemma* (New York: Penguin, 2006), on a tour of a well-run plant. They were expecting to witness all the horrors, but they were sur-

prised to learn of the operator's sincere desire to do the job properly. I doubt if we will soon achieve a switch from this system of processing and distribution to the ideal of sustainable farming, which
includes raising animals the organic way. Some of the fight for a better system must be directed to legislators. Meanwhile, look for the
cleanest and most humane source of meat available for your family's consumption.

- Real meat-eating is neither easy nor is it any guarantee of longevity. The cheetah is just about the fastest land predator there is,
but fewer than a third of their young reach adulthood, and those
that do live only about seven years. Vegetarian elephants and tor-
toises live between 70 and 150 years.

- Spend a while with a baby calf. Once one of the little critters sucks
on your finger, you will think twice about your next pot roast.

- Here's what did it for me: in 1974, I watched a flock of blood-
soaked vultures attack an enormous pile of intestines and skin
rotting in the sun near a West African open-air meat market. The
smell was pretty memorable, too.

- Mad cow disease. Ever hear of "mad vegetable disease"?

- We kill 100,000 head of cattle for food every day, just to supply
the United States. Worldwide, it is a bovine holocaust.

- The pig population in North Carolina produces as much sewage
as the entire human population of New York City.[8]

- "Emu Meat Now for Sale": I do not doubt the culinary experience
of Australia's gastronomic experts, but when somebody tells me
of the advantages of emu flesh, all I think of are five-foot-high
birds with dust-mop feathers, big round eyes, four-inch beaks,
and ravenous appetites. I don't think I could bring myself to eat
emu, even though it would serve them right, as I was ungraciously
harassed by a renegade flock of them in Canberra, Australia.

- Of 2,000 workers at one meatpacking plant, 800 became disabled in one year.[9]

- Chicken shades: Hens by the thousands are raised in such claustrophobic, crowded cages that the birds will actually peck each other to death. To reduce aggression in chickens, red-tinted contact lenses are now marketed for poultry workers to slip into the birds' eyes.

How to Moderate Your Meat Intake

On the farm, I (AWS) got to know a lot of calves. One was born literally while the mother cow was making her way into the barn. In less than ten minutes, he was up and walking around. At the end of the day, I saw him in the pasture, following his mother; he took about ten steps to her one. Of course, the future for male bovines was bleak: females would live to become milkers, but the boys would become veal.

"Veal" has big brown eyes with long, delicate lashes. "Veal" will suck on your fingers thinking you are its mother. "Veal" is kept in horrible, cramped pens, some so small that the calf cannot even turn around. Calves are loaded with antibiotics to keep them alive. A day or two after birth, they are taken from their mother and fed artificial milk replacer. Mom goes into the milking line to provide for our breakfast, not to feed her baby.

The calf is sent to slaughter for your next order of veal parmesan. There is a way to stop it: eliminate the demand. If we do not eat veal, calves will not be killed. If we do not eat meat, steers will not be killed. Reducing the demand is almost as good: less is better for them; less is healthier for you. And "less" is eminently doable.

I (RC) have to admit that I, too, suffer from the "Bambi connection"—those big brown eyes can disturb your heart. After having deer adopt my orchard for their winter headquarters and chomping up everything green (and even "deer-proofed") including thirty-year-old landscaping, I get a little fire in my eyes. I feel that with only the slightest suggestion a sensitive five-year-old can make the connection that he is eating a once life-loving, happy-go-lucky animal. I heard

4-H advisors tell their future farmers and ranchers to not make the mistake of putting a name to their animal project. Advertisers of eggs from "free-range chickens" often don't fully describe the range that their "happy" chickens roam, although these conditions from both a health and a humane treatment standpoint are infinitely better than the way most are raised.

PASS THE MUSTARD, OR JUST PASS ON THE HOT DOG?

More hot dogs are eaten at the Fourth of July holiday than at any other time of the year. The National Hot Dog and Sausage Council states that "during the Independence Day weekend, 155 million will be gobbled up" and that Americans consume more than 7 billion hot dogs over the summer. Americans eat an average of sixty hot dogs each per year.[10]

Is a hot dog or two a week a big deal? Perhaps it is. Children who eat one hot dog a week double their risk of a brain tumor; two per week triples the risk. Kids eating more than twelve hot dogs a month (three a week) have nearly ten times the risk of leukemia as children who eat none.[11] And it is not just about kids: of 190,000 adults studied for seven years, those eating the most processed meat, such as deli meats and hot dogs, had a 68 percent greater risk of pancreatic cancer than those who ate the least.[12]

Think twice before you serve up your next hot dog. If your family is going to eat hot dogs, at least take your vitamins. Hot dog–eating children taking supplemental vitamins were shown to have a reduced risk of cancer.[13] Vitamins C and E prevent the formation of nitrosamines, potentially cancer-causing compounds found in preserved meat products.[14]

Any meat that has to rely on artificial redness provided by unhealthy nitrites and artificial coloring should be scorned. When a child is old enough to understand why Mom was so mean by not letting him freely indulge, there can be an early lesson of accepting responsibility for one's own health.

Dr. Lendon Smith, the well-known pediatrician and author of *Feed Your Kids Right,* speaks of non-foods or bad foods as "antinutrients." As such, they are simply to be left out of the picture. A parent offers a new food that has his or her approval. As the child gains under-standing, there is room for negotiation. To avoid "food fights," be aware of how an intelligent toddler loves to manipulate the diet over-seer and exercise power: "You can't make me eat." Good attitudes about foods should begin early. If opportunities were missed, expect a transition period of as long as two months for change to take hold.

WHAT ABOUT DAIRY FOODS?

Relatively few people have ready access to fresh, raw milk. I (AWS) personally think that cheese and yogurt have a place in a healthy, natural diet for a child. To me, dairy is a better choice than meat. Again speaking as a former dairyman, I'd rather milk a cow than kill one. But that also means the milk should be fresh and minimally processed, not the skimmed, pasteurized, hormone-laden, antibiotic-ridden, hyper-allergenic white water that passes for "milk" nowadays. I support the use of scrupulously clean, unpasteurized ("raw") milk. As a dairyman, I raised my family on unpasteurized milk from cows I knew rather intimately. I milked 120 cows, twice a day, with the help of a small but modern milking parlor. I kept their quarters clean and their milk clean. Clean, healthy cows give clean, healthy milk.

There are some farms that I would not knowingly drink milk from, cooked or not. Since most consumers have no choice and no infor-mation as to just whose milk is in the carton, pasteurization is an attempt to reduce bacteria count from the sloppiest farms. Pasteur-ization temperatures are not hot enough to do the job properly, and high-temperature autocleaving destroys nutritional value. I think we would do a lot better to focus on farm sanitation.

I raised my kids as lacto-ovo-vegetarians and they are now tall, strong adults. Elephants never eat eggs or dairy, and they are even taller and stronger. Kids can get protein and calcium (the usual rea-sons, aside from taste, that people choose to eat dairy products) from foods other than milk and eggs. If you check a nutrition textbook or online nutrition tables, you will see that beans, whole-grain breads, and even vegetables have significant amounts of protein.

Some people do much better with no dairy or eggs whatsoever. For example, pasteurized-milk allergies appear to be very common in children. They have been linked with sinus problems, diabetes, constipation and diarrhea, chronic ear infections, behavior problems, and asthma.[15] I think that, in many cases, these symptoms are often due to overall poor diet and vitamin deficiencies and are then greatly aggravated by consuming milk. If one is allergic to milk (pasteurized is more of a culprit than raw), there are symptoms. If not allergic to milk, the symptoms either are not there or are due to other more obscure causes.

- Constipation is easy to cure and uncomplicated diarrhea can be kept in check with initial fasting, judicious use of cultured milk products (cheese and yogurt), and plenty of daily fiber.

- Behavior problems need modification therapy and megavitamin therapy, heavy on the niacin.[16] The why's and how's are addressed in Chapters 10 and 11.

- Earaches and ear infections can be obliterated with vitamin C. Vitamin C therapy is discussed in Chapter 12. First of all, be sure to get at the underlying cause. Some children with recurrent ear infections do vastly better with a reduction in dairy products. We think all do better with good, wholesome diet, low on sugar and virtually free of junk food.

An unusually restricted diet for your kids can backfire on you. I have seen a few scrawny vegan children in my time, and I have also seen a large number of obese, meat-fattened children. You simply must keep a reasonable eye on your kids' diet. This may sound rather odd: you need to be an extremist, but moderately so. This does not mean "in all things, moderation" but rather "in unimportant things, flexibility." Both over-compliance and under-compliance can result in a sick child. Hold firm on what is important: eating right every day, exercising regularly, taking supplements, avoiding chemical additives and pesticides, and taking charge of your own health. Stick to the main points; compromise on the minor points. Health is and always will be about balanced living.

There will be times when you need a doctor. Let's hope a balance can be found between standard medicine and orthomolecular medicine, by having parents and doctors listen to each other. There are children's doctors who can overcome the limiting effects of our health-care system. They are as willing to learn from you as you are from them. Seek them out.

SUMMARY

Who will decide when experts disagree? Well, practically no one agrees on all aspects of every diet. It's like your grandmother probably said: "Don't talk about religion or politics at the dinner table." And if you talk too much about the dinner itself, or worry too much about everything, eating is no fun. So, use your good sense and read about others' good sense. Really think about what you feed your kids before you set the table, even before you shop for groceries. Do the best you can and follow these general rules:

- Eat whole, unprocessed foods.

- Do not eat junk food.

- Avoid sugar.

- Do not overdo it on meat.

- Eat lots of fruits and vegetables, raw when possible.

- Dairy products are generally good, but not for all people. See what works best for your family.

- Eggs are good for you. Try to buy organic eggs and make sure they are as fresh as possible.

- Butter is better than any of the fake yellow spreads available.

- When you sit down to a meal, enjoy it!

CHAPTER 6

CHILDREN AND CHOLESTEROL

"I find medicine is the best of all trades because whether you do any good or not you still get your money."
—MOLIÈRE, *THE DOCTOR IN SPITE OF HIMSELF* (1664)

Childhood obesity has reached epidemic proportions in the United States, more than tripling in the last three decades. The prevalence of obesity among children and adolescents is nearly 20 percent, and rising. What could have a more devastating impact on kids' health? Obesity makes it more likely that these children suffer from heart disease, high blood pressure, diabetes, bone and joint problems, and social and psychological problems.[1]

Obesity is multifactorial, including genetic, behavioral, and environmental factors. Caloric imbalance (expending too few calories for the amount of calories consumed), poor diet, and lack of physical activity are important considerations. "Childhood obesity is almost completely preventable," states cardiologist Dean Ornish, M.D. "We don't have to wait for a new drug or technology; we just have to put into practice what we already know. What's changed is our diet and lifestyle. If we caused it, we can reverse it."[2] Consider this: a typical teenage boy drinks 20 ounces of sugary soda a day. Experts agree that Americans' increasingly sedentary lifestyle and fondness for fast food has contributed to our increasing girth.

Thus, it is a bit of a shock to see conventional medicine recommend cholesterol-lowering drugs such as Lipitor for children. The emphasis on cholesterol in the diet as a cause for heart disease—an idea clung to for decades by media and medicine alike—turned out to be a myth. Yet, the American Academy of Pediatrics (AAP), which has 60,000 pediatrician members, has said that it wants kids as young as eight years of age to take cholesterol-lowering drugs.[3] One should keep in mind that the AAP administers projects that receive cash from drug companies, including PediaMed, McNeil, Sanofi-Aventis, AstraZeneca, Dermik, Abbott, and Merck.[4] The AAP also receives money from Pepsi and McDonalds.[5]

Side effects of cholesterol-lowering drugs include fever, liver damage, muscle pain, rhabdomyolysis (muscle breakdown), memory loss, personality changes, irritability, headaches, anxiety, depression, chest pain, acid regurgitation, dry mouth, vomiting, leg pain, insomnia, eye irritation, tremors, dizziness, and more.

The AAP is wrong to advocate drug therapy for obese children. Cardiovascular disease is not caused by a failure to take enough pharmaceuticals as a child—it is a lifestyle disease. Kids need to eat right and exercise. If they need help lowering cholesterol, give them a safe vitamin, not a drug, and urge them to eat healthier and exercise more.

WHAT IS CHOLESTEROL?

Cholesterol is not a fat but a huge alcohol that combines with fatty acids to produce a cholesterol ester. It has twenty-seven carbons in four carbon rings. Cholesterol is found in bile and makes up gallstones. Natural body steroids ("fat-related compounds"), such as sex hormones, vitamin D, and adrenal hormones, are cholesterol-based. Steroids, by the way, come from sterols, which are large, many-ringed alcohols. Coenzyme Q_{10} (valuable in energy production) and the other fat-soluble vitamins—A, E, and K—are derived from precursors of cholesterol itself.

Cholesterol is essential to life, specifically in cell membranes, brain, and nerve tissue. It is made by the body (endogenous supply), mostly in the liver, and occurs only in animal foods (meat, eggs, dairy); plants, and their oils, do not contain any. If you never ate any cholesterol, your body would still make plenty. This is a strong argument for avoiding it. If an infant is fed formula that is too low in cholesterol, its body will get into a pattern of cholesterol overproduction by the liver.

Cholesterol must be put into a water-soluble form in order to be transported in the bloodstream. This is done through a complex molecule called a lipoprotein, which consists of four parts: a triglyceride, cholesterol, an apoprotein, and a phospholipid. The phospholipid has an emulsifying property that breaks up the larger fat particles.

When discussing "cholesterol," it usually is in reference to cholesterol as part of the lipoprotein. The lipoproteins are named according to their density. Protein is heavier than fat, so the lipoprotein with the greater protein-to-fat ratio is the more dense. The largest (less dense) cholesterol-containing fat particle is the chylomicron, which comes from the intestine shortly after a meal and goes directly through blood and lymph channels to muscle or fat tissue. After these tissues have their requirements met, the residue is transported to the liver by high-density lipoproteins (HDLs). In the liver, very-low-density lipoproteins (VLDLs) are formed, which contain 80 percent triglycerides (fats with three carbon atoms).

The fatty acids are either saturated or polyunsaturated. The marbled fat of "choice" beef, and what we call the undesirable stuff in our bodies, is in a form of triglycerides with all three carbon sites occupied with saturated fats. The triglyceride molecule itself is not water soluble (it has to be part of the lipoprotein), but it is a form that can transport the fatty acids from the body of a cell into the "engines of the cell" (with the aid of another enzyme), after the lipoprotein gets them into the cell.

VLDLs are assembled in the liver and go to peripheral tissues, where they are degraded to intermediate-density lipoproteins (IDLs). This step and the next to low-density lipoprotein (LDL) formation get their cholesterol returned to the liver via HDLs. All of which is done within liver metabolism, with no further contribution from a dietary source. It should be emphasized that carbohydrate intake has a much greater effect on triglyceride production than dietary cholesterol. There are LDL receptors in other than liver tissues, which break down the complex lipoprotein. The cholesterol is either incorporated into the cell membrane or stored in the cell. An abundance, by acting through a limiting enzyme, suppresses synthesis (insulin stimulates it) and inhibits synthesis in receptors.

It should be noted that 80 percent of what we call cholesterol of measurable blood levels is produced in the liver, leaving only 20 percent derived from diet. A heavy dietary load suppresses cholesterol synthesis in the liver. When the components of a lipoprotein become oxidized, the potential for harmful health effects is greatly increased. Thus, the need for antioxidant vitamins, both water-soluble vitamin C and fat-soluble vitamin E, in optimal amounts to prevent oxidation.

When cholesterol-containing fatty deposits (plaques) build up in and on the walls of the arteries, the result is atherosclerosis. This process is often considered to be an underlying cause of heart disease. And it is true that high serum cholesterol levels are associated with atherosclerosis. The question is, what causes cholesterol to be deposited in the arteries? Vitamin C advocate and Nobel Prize–winner Linus Pauling thought it was a lack of vitamin C and the amino acid lysine. For many years, it has been widely recommended that everyone reduce daily cholesterol intake. It is even more important to increase dietary fiber, because fiber binds and helps eliminate bile acids, which contain cholesterol. Even just two medium-sized carrots a day will lower serum cholesterol by over 10 percent in just a few weeks. Oats, onions, cabbage, broccoli, beans, grapefruit, and apples work, too, because calcium pectate in these foods binds bile acids and reduces cholesterol absorption.

Why is cholesterol associated with atherosclerosis? When there is a break in the lining of an arterial wall, and adequate vitamin C is present, there is immediate healing. If not, plasminogen, a precursor of the "clot buster" plasmin, takes its place and prevents healing. Also, apolipoprotein(a), the apoprotein of a cholesterol-containing lipoprotein, stands in for vitamin C and takes its place to patch up the lesion, but in doing so, it forms what we call "plaque." This should be a good reason to have adequate amounts of vitamin C in your body at all times.

FAT PHOBIA

The past couple of decades have been the dark ages of overblown "fat phobia." Nevertheless, in spite of opposition, we have progressed from darkness into nutritional enlightenment. Simplistic, early thinking was that virtually all fat is bad—saturated fats, large amounts of polyunsaturated fats (including the essential fatty acids, without which good health is impossible), monounsaturated fats, and especially cholesterol. The much-advocated solution was to eliminate fat from the diet, or at least to reduce fat intake as much as possible.

Then, special attention was brought to bear on cholesterol over the other kinds of fats. The simplistic thinking went like this:

- Egg yolks contain cholesterol.

- Cholesterol is thought to cause "hardening of the arteries"—most dangerous in the coronary arteries that nourish the heart itself.

- Therefore, don't eat eggs (at first, not even the egg white).

A whole industry sprang up, and cholesterol testing went wild. Initially, attention was paid only to total blood levels of cholesterol. Slowly, there evolved a look at specific fractions, starting with separating LDLs from HDLs. LDL became known as "bad" cholesterol and HDL as "good" cholesterol, as it was felt that HDL helped transport cholesterol out of the body. Triglycerides gained prominence when they were recognized as precursors of LDLs.

The medical profession's zero tolerance for cholesterol and other fats was very harmful. Almost any food that tasted good was off limits. Eggs topped the list of bad foods, followed by butter, even though the "bad rap" could not be substantiated. Studies as far back as 1939 show little effect on blood cholesterol levels from a huge intake of egg yolks.[6] A high dietary intake of cholesterol has been shown to actually reduce endogenous production by the liver. An infant deprived of cholesterol in the formula early on will produce above normal levels of endogenous cholesterol.

Egg yolks have twice the content of the very important nutrient choline compared to the next best source, beef liver. (Since the liver of any animal collects, processes, and rids toxins from the body, liver is a very poor second to egg yolks.) Acetylcholine is the neurotransmitter that is deficient in Alzheimer's disease. A choline source not only supplies the choline for the neurotransmitter but also the chemical units called methyl groups that are an essential part of many enzyme systems. Egg yolks are a good source of many other nutrients, especially bioflavonoids (which contribute to the orange color of yolks), vitamin A and folic acid, and the minerals calcium, phosphorus, and zinc. They are a nearly complete food, lacking only in fiber.

The industry's response to "bad" cholesterol in egg yolks was to "scientifically" develop a yolk-free egg product sold as Egg Beaters. This was what Michael Pollan, in his book *In Defense of Food,* calls "nutritionism,"[7] food super science at its finest. There were no long-term human studies done before approval. A study published in *Pediatrics,* the journal of the AAP, showed photos of laboratory rats on a diet of Egg Beaters and the control rats on their regular diet. I had never seen a rattier looking rat than the one on the test diet. Recently, I searched the Internet for a description of the original Egg Beaters and could only find a large variety of "new and improved" versions: some with a dash of egg yolk (to provide real egg flavor); others with a variety of "healthful" nutrients derived from vegetables and herbs. The original was free of any trace of yolk.

Advice on cholesterol and eggs from the American Heart Association has progressed painfully slowly. It has evolved somewhat: from egg whites only to an occasional imbibing of the real thing.

Saturated Fats

Early in the fat fight, saturated fats, especially butter, were vilified. They so condemned butter that they overlooked the fact that its substitute, if it were to stay solid in stick form, would also be a saturated fat, albeit an artificial one. Margarine was concocted: it looked like butter and tasted a little bit like butter, and it was cheaper. This miracle of science consisted of taking a polyunsaturated fatty acid derived from a relatively cheap vegetable oil and hydrogenating it. Hydrogenation consists of artificially forcing hydrogen to "saturate" carbon-carbon double bonds. Why do it? In order to change the fat from a liquid at room-temperature into a butter-like solid, margarine. This creation, a trans-fat, was designed to prevent the development of rancidity, a result of oxidation. To further the look-alike image, early pale-white margarines included a little packet of coloring that, when stirred in, simulated the yellow of butter.

It has taken many years to discover that this scientifically designed substance would not be able to trick the body into believing it is the real thing. Our bodies are not designed to adequately metabolize this imposter. Dr. Walter Willet, Dean of Public Health at Harvard Medical School, has stated his belief that if we would ban trans-fats, as Denmark has done, it would be the equivalent of putting every American on a statin (cholesterol lowering) drug. He also believes that some of the bad press that saturated fats have been given is due to studies that don't split out trans-fats but include them along with natural saturated fats.[8]

Essential Fatty Acids

During the "all fats are bad" initial era, even essential fatty acids (EFAs) were included. The new term, fatty acids, was not well received by a subculture that didn't like the connotations of either "fatty" or "acid." Like vitamins, the basic omega-6 fatty acid (precursor to the fatty acids of vegetable oils) and the basic omega-3 fatty acid (precursor to fish oils) are called "essential" because they truly are. Our bodies can build on these essentials to form the longer-chain fatty acids that function to either promote or reduce inflammation (among other benefits). But the essential building blocks must come from dietary intake.

The "no fat" campaign was so effective that a mother I saw during a well-baby check challenged me after I told her that skim milk was not for infants. The infant was terribly scrawny and malnourished, with scaly and dry skin, typical of essential fatty acid deprivation. It was also irritable, likely due to nutrient starvation. I pointed out all these signs to the mother, who then told me in no uncertain

FATS AND APPETITE SUPPRESSION

Fats have a marvelous way of staying in the stomach for longer periods than carbohydrates, which provides a feeling of satiety. Butter also has the quality of adding enjoyable flavor to a food (just consult any Julia Child cookbook). Making butter a bad actor along with all its relatives overlooked its uniqueness. Its short-chain fatty acid, butyric acid, encourages the growth of favorable bacteria (probiotics) in the gut, which, among many other functions, synthesize a portion of the B vitamin pyridoxine (B_6). This should get one thinking more about quality rather than simply quantity, and incorporating saturated fats in the diet without over-indulging.

terms that I was ignorant and should get with the program, because all other doctors were continually saying that fat is bad.

Polyunsaturated Fats

Eventually, polyunsaturated fats were ushered in as substitutes for animal (saturated) fats. Most any polyunsaturated fat would do, and trans-fats were somehow mentally mingled with natural vegetable oils. Presumably since they started life as polyunsaturated fatty acids, they could still fall into that category. There are studies supporting the lowering of cholesterol levels with polyunsaturated fatty acids, but these designed studies exclude "confounding factors" such as trans-fats and select out certain fats. Studies done on a general population don't share that sophistication. How can the dietary ratio of omega-6 to omega-3 fatty acids be determined in a random population that is ignorant of these designations?

Dietary long-chain fatty acids are contained in oils commonly thought of as either vegetable oils or fish oils. While the EFAs are ingested from the diet, the long-chain fatty acids can be made in the body if certain vitamin cofactors are present. Still, there is individual variability in this synthesis, so eating the final product is a more certain way of getting a sufficient amount. A fat with only one number attached is actually a composite of other types of fatty acids but is named for the predominating one. Wheat germ is predominately an omega-6 (50 percent) but also contains omega-3s, monounsaturated fats, and saturated fatty acids.

Some of these long-chain polyunsaturated acids are contained in cell walls in the form of prostaglandins. Prostaglandins are like hormones that are released upon demand. Some, mainly the omega-6-derived prostaglandins, are noted for influencing inflammation, making platelets stick together, and promoting clot formation, while omega-3-derived prostaglandins have opposite functions.

Red Meat

Red meat was on the same hit list as fat due to its fat content. In this country, we take cattle off of natural grass pastures and transport them to a feedlot, crowd them together, and feed them omega-6-rich grains (mainly corn). The cattlemen are paid on the basis of overall weight of each head of cattle, whether the weight comes from fat or muscle. Fat is easier, quicker, and cheaper to produce. This was accommodated and encouraged by the U.S. Department of Agriculture's grading system of meat based on "marbling" (visible hard fat), the top grade being "choice." The fat of grass-fed cattle is abundant in polyunsaturated omega-3 fatty acids, while the grain-fed fat has more omega-6 fatty acids. Thus, grass-fed beef is a healthier choice. Furthermore, crowding in feedlots has necessitated antibiotic use in cattle to curtail the spread of bacterial infections. The causes of infection, and the dirty word itself, are glossed over, and antibiotics are now considered as weight-producing agents.

Carbohydrates

The next phase of poor advice on fat was the "pasta movement": shunning red meat and embracing carbohydrates. Any carbohydrate was recommended, simply because it differed from red meat or other "bad" fat, nutrient-rich animal sources. Of course, overconsumption of carbohydrates virtually guarantees obesity.

HYPOGLYCEMIA: ALL IN THE FAMILY

Hypoglycemia may have a familial basis, and this is easily observed in the "fight or flight" effect of adrenaline—the jitteriness, the manifestation of anxiety or mental fuzziness, or being in a "cold sweat." Hypoglycemia can be confirmed by a glucose tolerance test, in which a measured dose of glucose is given by mouth. Blood levels are tested periodically to note when a plunge in the blood glucose level occurs and how deep it is. A dip in glucose levels can start as soon as fifteen minutes or as late as two hours after the start of the test. Any degree of a hypoglycemic reaction should be noted, since it can affect mental function and behavior (attention deficit is a good example). Simple observation is often all that is necessary to diagnose all but the worst cases of hypoglycemia. Management if this condition should include:

- Imbibing sugars and refined starches cautiously.

- Accompanying sugars with fiber, fat, or protein to slow the process of glucose assimilation into the bloodstream.

- Thinking about when the next meal is due when a child is "out of fuel" (learn to recognize the individual signs, such as when a whiney child "collapses" and completely "loses it"). If mealtime is just around the corner, a bit of fruit juice might be in order. If mealtime is not due for some time (over half an hour), the juice alone could cause a cycle of improvement followed by another plunge. Then, the remedy is to follow the juice with a source of protein, fat, or both. My favorites include cheddar cheese, nuts, or sunflower seeds.

Popular carbohydrates were the high-glycemic index foods: white flour, white rice, potatoes, sugar, and high-fructose corn syrup, which was coming into widespread use. The glycemic index is a measure of how quickly a food's glucose enters the bloodstream. Food starch consists of glucose molecules linked together in a chain that, upon digestion, readily breaks down again into glucose, putting the simple starch on par with sugars. When glucose enters the bloodstream, the pancreas releases insulin, which is needed to convert glucose to a form that can be used for energy production. After energy needs are met, insulin acts as a storage hormone, and excess glucose is converted to fat and enters the fat cells of our bodies. In primitive times, when food was scarce, this fat storage was a way to put energy producers in the bank to be drawn on in lean times.

Ingesting too much of a quickly assimilated glucose (or other sugars) causes the pancreas to release an abundance of insulin. This "overkill" of insulin is manifest when a "counterattack" from the hormone adrenaline kicks in. Paradoxically, this surge of too much glucose leads to hypoglycemia (too little). Insulin causes glucose blood levels to fall, but since brain metabolism is essentially dependent on glucose, adrenaline sets off a low-glucose alarm, and additional stores are released from other tissues or more is produced in the liver. If other food components (protein, fiber, fat) are ingested at the same time as a simple sugar or starch, the reaction is slowed and moderate amounts of high-glycemic foods do not set off this insulin overreaction.

Little by little, the folly of substituting refined carbohydrates for fats is being recognized. Articles suggesting that refined carbohydrates may have a more profound health effect than cholesterol are appearing in the medical literature. Also, there is more media exposure of the dangers of sugar, high-fructose corn syrup, and white flour. Increasing numbers of people are curtailing the use of these nutrient-free substances.

Whole-grain pasta is available and makes a desirable food. Soft drinks can and should be eliminated or greatly curtailed, especially in children. Even healthful fruit juices should be given in moderation (because of high levels of fruit sugars) and taken with something that sticks to the ribs.

SUMMARY

Nutrition advice from mainstream medicine has been dismal, and buying into it has steered us away from the road to health. Slowly but positively, attention is getting off of cholesterol and turning to the true nutritional bad actors. We have been misled into believing that it is the fat in our diet that translates directly to fat in our bodies. The real villain is refined carbohydrates that are doubly bad because they are nearly devoid of nutritional value.

We have pharmaceutical and food industries that bombard us with misinformation (and many times, lies). It is a shame that advertisements for cholesterol-lowering drugs are allowed. After one sees the guy who, "when diet and exercise weren't enough," got a prescription for the drug, followed by a quick spoken list of potential side effects, then comes the advice to "Ask your doctor." Turn up the volume when you get to the side effects, and you will likely totally reject the drug.

There has to be another way, and there is: the diet and vitamin supplement way. It worked for generations before our diets changed so radically. If you don't eat cholesterol, you'll make more of it in your body. Eggs and butter are good for your kids, always have been, always will be. Sedentary lifestyles, junk food, vitamin deficiency, and rampant sugar overdose are the real problems. Whole foods, supplements, and exercise are the solution. Feed those kids right and send them out to play!

CHAPTER 7

A TOXIC ENVIRONMENT AND WHAT TO DO ABOUT IT

*"Health is the finally effective test of the interaction of
the human organism with its total environment."*
—SCOTT NEARING, AUTHOR OF *LIVING THE GOOD LIFE*

We hear much about many obviously toxic things in our environment, such as agricultural chemicals and heavy metals, ending up in or on our bodies from our food and water, or in the air we breathe. Even many things alleged to be good for us—taking medicines, drinking eight glasses of water a day, eating fruits and vegetables, and indulging in outdoor aerobic exercise—may demand a closer look. Investigation should lead to realistic findings and, we hope, not to pessimism.

As soon as we discover that what we put in our mouths or breathe may be laced with hidden toxins, we have our work cut out for us. We need to know where toxins reside, what are the relevant determinations of toxic levels, what problems they pose, and how to avoid exposure or minimize the effects of exposure when it can't be avoided.

Our efforts won't noticeably change the big picture of an imperfect world, but we must continue to make inroads of positive change. We will first identify the main culprits. We will also describe some specific "vitamin cures" but mostly will emphasize the role of vitamins as preventive agents for prospective mothers, infants, and children, in order to minimize the impact of environmental toxins.

PESTICIDES AND INSECTICIDES

Pesticides

Finally, after a generation of widespread use of toxic pesticides, agriculture experts are beginning to recommend replacing some harmful pesticides with less toxic ones. They also are taking a closer look at better, safer agricultural practices, and listening to advocates of organic, sustainable farming.

In the Dust Bowl days of the Great Depression in the 1930s, great chunks of land were given to tough survivors as an incentive to stay put and attempt rejuvenation of the devastated grassy plains by "scientifically" raising an economically rewarding crop. Thousands of acres were devoted to a single crop, wheat. We know now what happens over time in a monoculture farming system: a decreased resistance to pests. Crop losses due to pests and the freeing up of the petroleum scarcity at the end of World War Two converged, which allowed for the development of chemical pesticides.

Poison gases used in warfare were designed to be nerve gases, toxic by contact with skin and mucous membranes and the respiratory tree. It was felt that insects would be more susceptible to the killing effect than humans. Basically, it was the simplistic thinking that went along the lines of using a tiny amount of what will kill big organisms to kill tiny organisms. Chemical derivatives of these war gases were developed and accepted as a standard part of new "scientific" farming practices. Chemical fertilizers were promoted as essential for large-scale farming. There was a linear correlation of pounds of applied nitrogen to pounds of yield. Pesticide use meant less of the harvest was sacrificed to pests: a boost for yields equated to more dollars of profits in the pockets of farmers.

Yield is a very tangible measure, but the undesirable side effects of chemical farming are difficult to evaluate, particularly in the short-term. For example, a suspected carcinogen (cancer-causing substance) could require as long as thirty years time to show its deleterious effects, from the first insult to a cell's DNA until a cancer has grown to detectable levels. In the class of pesticides called organophosphates, blood and urine samples may not reveal abnormally high levels because the chemical is hiding in fatty tissues. At the cellular level, we do not know what concentration is needed to initiate genetic damage or the significance of cumulative exposure.

The organophosphates are known to inhibit the enzyme cholinesterase, which normally breaks down the neurotransmitter acetylcholine instantly. Normally, if acetylcholine lingers too long at the interconnecting nerve junctions, the victim has trouble seeing due to "pin-point" pupils, develops a headache, becomes shaky, and may go on to convulsions, coma, and death. Alzheimer's disease manifestations are thought to be due to *inadequate* levels of acetylcholine, and one of the most popular drugs works by the same biochemistry as this group of pesticides. By inhibiting the enzyme cholinesterase, the drug allows acetylcholine–which is in short supply in Alzheimer's –to have a longer effect before it is broken down. Fortunately, many of the organophosphate pesticides have recently been banned and replaced with safer substances, thanks in part to the organic movement. Unfortunately, the banned pesticides may be sold to countries that have weak environmental laws.

Often, there are strong ties between farm chemical companies and land grant universities. If a question of a pesticide being the cause of cancer or a neurological disease should arise, the "expert testimony" for the manufacturer often is from a university agriculture professor. This arrangement can result in a nearly impenetrable defense. Add to this the difficulty of "proving" the cause of a disease that might develop over a period of many years and may have multiple causes.

A Case in Point

I (RC) would like to illustrate the far-reaching effects of this arrangement with a story from my own experience. Our county health department in Montana used to visit a nearby pristine area to provide health screenings and immunizations to school-aged children. The young families, by their own choosing, lived almost a pioneer existence. These visits established rapport and resulting trust. In May 1978, one of the young women confided to us that she had miscarried during the first trimester of her pregnancy. She soon discovered that seven other women in this small community had suffered a similar fate. We developed a questionnaire that included every possible cause of spontaneous abortion we could think of: description of diet, any medications, illnesses before or during the brief pregnancy, chemical exposures, source of drinking water, and so on. The personal interviews brought to light a commonality of headaches, starting with exposure to roadside spraying of herbicide and, for several, continuing throughout the short pregnancy. Later, one of the women found out that an unusually high concentration of the herbicide 2,4-dichlorophenoxyacetic acid (2,4-D) had been applied to their roadside the previous summer, probably by accident. Some family milk cows had been seen poking their heads through the fence and grazing on contaminated grass. The irony of all this was that the chosen lifestyle of the inhabitants had backfired. They raised their own vegetables, their meat was wild game, and they wanted their children to be raised in as pure an environment as possible, removed from city life.

Our story caught the eye of a local journalist, who got it into local newspapers. From there, a national news syndicate picked it up and spread the word nationwide. I was so surprised to get correspondence from all over the country telling me of individual and group efforts to get more attention paid to the known cancer-causing effects of this herbicide. As a result of the publicity, all sorts of "problems" evolved. The state toxicology laboratory suddenly didn't have the ability to analyze the frozen liver of the butchered milk cow. The women resided on both sides of a county line, making a legal "venue" impossible to determine. Organizations favoring the use of this popular herbicide, such as the state department of agriculture, pesticide manufacturers and distributors, and, sadly enough, even the state health department, quickly became very defensive and thwarted investigative efforts.

Dr. Bert Pfeiffer, a professor at the University of Montana who had investigated the effects of Agent Orange on the Vietnamese population, provided us with important information. Agent Orange was a combination of two herbicides, 2,4-D and 2,4,5-trichlorophenoxyacetic acid (2,4,5-T). They cause desiccation of plants by accelerating their growth to the point that the excessive growth rate and increased appetite outstrip the supply of soil nutrients, and plants starve to death. Toxic products called dioxins are associated mainly with 2,4, 5-T but can be found even with the more common 2,4-D, especially if it is exposed to high temperatures. Dioxins are among the most potent poisons known to humans. Medical conditions related to Agent Orange exposure included birth defects, a horrible skin condition called chloracne, and aplastic anemia (an often fatal condition in which the bone marrow stops making blood cells). These were early-onset effects, more easily correlated with dioxin exposure than are tumor-forming cancers. In spite of this knowledge, the herbicides of Agent Orange, under the trade name Silvex, continued to be approved for use in forested areas until Silvex was banned in 1984. 2,4-D has remained a widely used herbicide, even though there is much documentation on its relationship to cancer and blood dyscrasias (disorders), which is now easy to access on the Internet.

Before our county's weed-control warriors went forth to do battle against noxious roadside weeds, I attempted to arm them with knowledge of their "ordnance." I encouraged them to pay attention to what the manufacturer said regarding harmful side effects.. I gave clear explanations of how extra protection during the spray season, in the form of additional oral antioxidants, would help. We have much more to do in getting the toxicity message across. Nevertheless, my talks proved pretty ineffective, as I saw a county applicator spraying pesticides with no protective clothing and no mask (how could he wear a mask and keep his cigarette going?), with a breeze blowing this foul substance back on to him.

2,4-D is now being added to household lawn fertilizers in order to produce a "perfect" lawn. Personally, I have never objected to dandelions in a healthy lawn. With proper watering and other lawn health care, that splash of contrasting yellow will soon disappear. Children or pets should cancel one's plans for perfection anyway: it is a bad idea to put a carcinogen on a surface on which bare feet or bare paws come into contact. A local veterinarian, who is aware of this hazard, has found six cases of lymphoma in dogs.

Our county is home to seed potato production. Every effort is made to raise the best, disease-free potatoes, and an early frost is a great aid to harvest by shriveling the vines. Use of herbicides has now replaced this practice, as it was more predictable. The reputation of 2,4-D suffered around here when drifting from aerial application wiped out home garden tomato plants.

Although 2,4-D is still widely used, its popularity has been usurped by Roundup. Roundup is used on genetically engineered farm crops or on weeds around the house. The active ingredient, glyphosate, inhibits an enzyme involved in forming some essential amino acids. This mechanism of action is claimed to be peculiar to plants, so as not to affect the similar enzyme in mammals. However, Roundup also has been found to prevent binding of an ingredient to the active site of a core enzyme in all organisms.[1]

Much of the toxicity of Roundup is attributed to the surfactant added to the glyphosate and to the synergistic effect of the two ingredients. A surfactant is a substance that aids in getting the active ingredient where it is needed, such as sticking to foliage. This surfactant has been found to decrease RNA synthesis, delay embryonic development, and act synergistically with glyphosate.[2] There has been noted an association of Roundup with multiple myeloma (sometimes called bone cancer due to its destructive action on bone), and with non-Hodgkin's lymphoma.[3] Virtually no studies of the effects of Roundup on humans have been done. In time, when Roundup has as long a track record as 2,4-D, I think we might see similar associations. Multiple myeloma and embryonic abnormalities are representative of more active tissues being exposed and will reveal their pathology sooner after exposure than with most cancers.

The bigger hazard comes from the use of Roundup Ready, a system of genetically engineered seed that is resistant to the herbicide. Theoretically, then, Roundup can be used on the protected crop with impunity while killing all surrounding weeds. The manufacturer, Monsanto, owns the seed—considered "intellectual property"—and can sue a farmer trying to save seed for the next year's planting. According to a report from the Union of Concerned Scientists in 2004, the Roundup Ready system worked as promised for only three years before weed resistance occurred. For a replacement for

Roundup-resistant weed control, even more toxic herbicides like Atrazine were used, a poor choice as it is strongly associated with harm to embryos and already banned in Europe. Control of the spread of Roundup Ready genes to neighboring conventional crops has not been attained as promised. Reports of massive crop failures from its use rarely are revealed to the public, but they have occurred. Studies show great toxicity to earthworms and freshwater fish by run-off from cropland contaminated with Roundup. Still, more is being used on the top genetically engineered crops: corn, soybeans, and cotton. By 2005, 85 percent of soybeans in the U.S. were grown with this system, and soy products end up in the oil, flour, and lecithin in processed foods.

We have enough of a problem controlling this toxic substance getting *on* our food crops, but problems are multiplied by allowing it *in* our food supply. One doesn't normally think of cotton as a food crop, but cottonseed oil, along with soybean oil, is found in many processed foods, often as trans-fats (or "hydrogenated vegetable oil"). Regulatory bodies are reluctant to label genetically engineered foods, so consumers have no way of knowing if what they purchase is truly safe. At present, only certified organic foods are labeled to assure that they are pesticide free. Otherwise, we need to be vigilant of other genetically engineered foods entering the food supply.

Insecticides

The most famous (or infamous) killer of insects was the chlorinated hydrocarbon DDT (dichlorodiphenyltrichloroethane), a nerve gas derivative. Prior to its development, two "natural" pesticides, rotenone and pyrethrum, were the only options. Pyrethrum is derived from a flower of the chrysanthemum genus. Because of low immediate toxicity and the fact that it is biodegradable, it has stood the test of time. Rotenone, made from certain roots, is quite safe in the concentrations in which it is used. It works both by contact and ingestion, so it was used more for caterpillar, spider and mite eradication. World War Two interfered with the availability of these products, prompting the development of the synthetic DDT. It was chosen by the belief that while it was a very effective insect killer, it posed a relatively low hazard to warm-blooded animals.

The first real challenge to synthetic pesticide use came from the groundbreaking book *Silent Spring* by Rachel Carson, published in 1962. Carson had previously written extensively as a marine biologist and then turned her attention to environmental problems related to pesticide use. In her book, she expressed concern about bioaccumulation and the chemical industry's spreading of "disinformation." She described poisoning from pesticides and their relationship to cancer, and she accurately predicted that pest resistance would appear along with the advent of invasive species. Carson advocated biological control of pests, such as competing species, in place of pesticides. *Silent Spring* kicked off a groundswell of what came to be called the "environmental movement," leading to the formation of the Environmental Protection Agency (EPA).

Persistence in the environment and accumulation in the fatty tissues of mammals were two important characteristics of DDT and of others in this class that were developed later. It took time for these characteristics to become apparent. Meanwhile, environmentalists discovered the effects of DDT on the eggs of predator birds: eggshells were often too thin to support the life of developing birds. Mother birds had been feeding in areas where DDT had been sprayed many years before. Measurements of DDT levels in fatty tissues of numerous species yielded high readings. As is often the case, we show more concern for birds and whales than we do for human safety, but eventually attention shifted to related health problems in humans. In relating toxic effects from farm chemicals to cancer and other disorders, we get a more assured relationship with diseases that develop rapidly and bypass the silent latent period that may span many years. As with 2,4-D, the leukemias, aplastic anemia, and some lymphomas have a clear connection with these chlorinated hydrocarbons and the more widely used organophosphates.[4] Many studies support a connection between organophosphate pesticide exposure and Parkinson's disease.[5] There are some that see a more general relationship to other neurological diseases, such as Alzheimer's[6] and even attention deficit disorder.[7] I fear that seeking proof of *the* cause of these conditions that have unclear biochemical bases will allow us to keep our heads stuck in the sand.

Muddled jurisdiction between the U.S. Department of Agriculture and the EPA interferes with correcting the deficiencies in oversight. Lobbying by producers of farm chemicals, backed by "expert" advice, provide our legislators only with a biased point of view, not a good basis for lawmaking. For whatever reasons, the EPA is horribly behind in its safety testing of pesticides. A 2006 *Wall Street Journal* article told of EPA scientists blasting their superiors concerning the lack of toxicity testing for organophosphates.[8] The Food Quality Protection Act of 1996 required the agency to review acceptable limits of existing pesticides (specifically, those that attack the nervous system) within ten years. This wasn't done; neither were these replaced with safer chemicals. The article stated that the EPA was aware that some pesticides can easily enter the brain of fetuses and young children, but that they still lacked an evaluating procedure for testing toxicity to the nervous system. We simply have to employ self-help as we monitor the safety aspects of these chemicals.

What You Can Do About Pesticides and Insecticides

We have gone to some length describing the use and drawbacks of herbicides and the organophosphate pesticides. It is a lot easier to say, "Avoidance is the best policy" than to tell you how to do that. Consider increasing your intake of organic foods, which are healthy for you and the environment. However, we all have to consider cost and availability, and then compromise. Fortunately, there is an increasing demand for organic produce and more interest in the health advantages of locally grown produce. Demand doesn't necessarily equate to availability. The process of change is slow.

Dr. Bruce Ames, designer of the "Ames test" that determines the cancer-causing potential of chemicals,[9] also has done research on antioxidant levels in foods. At the time, I felt that he was selling out to the farm chemical industry when he stated that, due to the high antioxidant content of fruits and vegetables, we should eat more of them even when they are laced with pesticides. Since we can't, as of now, find ideal conditions, we will all have to do our best with what we have (but continuously push for the better).

In our favor, some toxic pesticides and fungicides have a short half-life and would leave very little residue on produce. Unfortunately, there is no way for the consumer to learn what chemicals were actually used. Using soap or detergent, we can often wash away much of the unknown residue. Water alone does nothing to dissolve or remove petrochemical pesticides. If you can, spend the extra money for organic foods that contain large amounts of phyto-antioxidants or other nutrients in their skin, which would be lost from peeling. Eggplant, red apples, and potatoes fall into that category. We don't eat banana skins, and there are other fruits that could be peeled without too much sacrifice of nutrition value. Blueberries are subjected to many farm chemicals, but dilute-soap washing will help a great deal. Perhaps, until better times, we will have to make the "Ames Compromise." These high-powered plant antioxidants were developed to protect the plant from pests. We should do the same by boosting our intake of these foods and by taking extra vitamin C, vitamin E, and the trace mineral selenium.

HEAVY METALS

Lead

Lead, of all the heavy metals, has occupied the number one spot in the pediatric medical literature. Some of the obvious signs and symptoms of acute lead poisoning have been known for a very long time. As with other environmental toxins, attempts to address the formation of safety standards for long-term exposure are not as straightforward.

Being anti-corrosive and malleable, lead has been smelted and used for thousands of years. A Roman engineer noted signs of toxicity and pronounced that he thought earthenware pipes would be safer than lead pipes for transporting water. Romans cooked in lead cookware and may have added a lead-containing substance to their wine—the kind of chronic exposure whose effects are harder to pin down. Toxicity was recognized in the 1600s in miners and smelter workers exposed to lead dust or fumes.

Occupational, acute exposure was the main focus until around 1897, when an Australian physician recognized the toxic effects from lead exposure in children. Recognition of the danger from leaded paint was discovered shortly thereafter; some countries banned lead paints as early as 1909. The League of Nations (a precursor to the United Nations) enacted a ban in 1922. By contrast, the United States did not start a ban until 1971, which didn't become complete until 1978.

Lead is very toxic and has a wide range of effects on the body and brain. As with other toxins, lead exposure hurts children sooner, and at lower doses. Acute symptoms will only be observed when the child has an exposure similar to the magnitude of an occupational exposure. The signs and symptoms produced by long-term exposure are milder and often indistinguishable from those attributed to other causes: diminished appetite, constipation, abdominal pain, irritability or lethargy, and anemia or kidney disease. Adults exhibit similar symptoms, but lead's effect on the nervous system is easier to define as they might include headache, tingling in the extremities, or feeling "fuzzy brained"—things that a young child can't describe. Workers in a plant that manufactured tetraethyl lead (TEL), the "anti-knock" gasoline additive, suffered from dementia and became known as "loony lead workers." Since young nervous systems are more prone to damage, it has become essential that we seek out the sources of lead exposure and find a more precise, acceptable blood level for children. Besides leaded paint, TEL has been the biggest lead disrupter of a child's nervous system: paint by ingestion of paint chips; TEL by breathing fumes.

In a gasoline-powered engine, if some gas ignites prematurely, the explosion driving the piston down is inefficient and causes a "knock." So General Motors, among others, developed TEL, which slowed the burn a bit and was defined as an anti-knock substance. When added to gasoline, the final product was simply called "ethyl." Ethyl came on the market in the early 1920s, and early on, extreme toxicity was discovered in TEL refinery workers. Public health experts warned the producers, but to no avail. The issue would not go away, so a conference was held in 1925 to look for alternative ways to improve fuel. Ethanol was examined but, in the amounts needed for effectiveness, it was determined (by the petroleum industry) that ethanol would be too costly. Furthermore, it was decided that the low levels of ethyl emitted from automobile exhaust were not a health hazard. Further research was funded by the lead industry. In 1943, a doctor equated behavior problems in children to lead exposure. When the issue went to court, it was the industry doctor's opinion that held sway.

The industry's safety assessment of TEL might have been adequate for the 1920s. Not that many vehicles were exhaling TEL in those days, but just think about the volume of exhaust gases produced every hour on or near a modern freeway. And consider the additional displacement of a modern car engine. Lettuce grown in fields adjacent to a freeway system was found to contain high levels of lead derived from TEL. A health hazard from this could be circumvented in iceberg lettuce by throwing away the outer leaves. Not so for more open leafy vegetables. This organic form of lead, being fat-soluble, gets past respiratory tract barriers and into the bloodstream more readily than the inorganic forms, such as lead dust or even smelter fumes.

After the qualms about lead toxicity effects in children were brushed aside in 1943, it wasn't until the 1970s that we got serious about lead exposure again, when articles by Herbert Needleman, M.D., started to appear in pediatric medical journals. Dr. Needleman conducted many of his own studies, and he garnered a lot of interest from his medical colleagues. This brought the focus back to evaluating the toxicity of TEL. The EPA finally began a ban on the additive in 1976 and it was completed in 1978, the same year as the ban on lead paint, catching up to what other civilized countries had already done.

Lead is a bad actor. It does mischief by binding to sulfur groups in some of our essential amino acids, the building blocks of proteins. Remember that enzymes that control our metabolic processes are made of proteins. Heme, the nucleus of hemoglobin that transports oxygen throughout our bodies, is very sensitive to lead. Anemia and a condition of red blood cells called basophilic stippling are the result.

Many other enzyme actions are fouled by lead. Interference with normal calcification of bone can be seen by a "lead line" near the growth plate of a large bone like the femur. This lead is sequestered in bone and is merely a marker of lead exposure, causing no harm. These are tangible findings along with measurement of lead concentration in hair, teeth, and nails. These findings represent low-dose, long-term exposure.

What needs to be determined is the lowest acceptable blood concentration that causes even minor brain damage. It is felt that lead interferes with synapse (the junction between nerve cells) formation, the development of neurotransmitters, and also causes loss of myelin sheaths. All of these effects can be manifest as behavior problems, even poorly defined ones such as attention deficit or aggressive behavior. Unlike a tangible laboratory test, behavior problems do not have such clear associations with a single cause. When a child's mental development is on the line, we will bend over backwards in our search for reliable safety standards, even without a proven association.

In 1970 the accepted maximum blood lead level was 60 mcg/dL (60 micrograms per tenth of a liter). In other words, a child with a level under 60 mcg/dL was considered healthy. Whether they were healthy or not was hardly ever verified. Between 1991 and 1994, when a standard of only 10 mcg/dL was in place, only 4.4 percent of children had a higher level, with 2–4 mcg/dL being the average. Getting TEL out of the environment was considered to be the biggest factor in the reduction. TEL, then, had proven to be the major source of children's lead exposure. So how do some have blood levels dangerously above the norm?

Even though leaded indoor paint was banned in 1978, many walls were still decorated with peeling, leaded paint years later. There was no edict demanding that landlords strip the paint off the walls in their rentals and repaint with safe material. It was in such dwellings, some of which were near the home of our legislators, that paint-eating toddlers were rediscovered. As soon as our legislators made the discovery, a nationwide hunt for high blood lead levels was launched.

Some state health programs balked at the idea of widespread screening with blood tests before narrowing the field by taking individual lead exposure history. A questionnaire might start by asking about symptoms of lead toxicity and then, in consideration of the most common cause, asking about evidence of eating peeling paint. Depending on the uniqueness of the area and its culture there would be questions pertaining to more rare exposure. Near the Mexican border one might ask a parent if they use imported ceramic cookware, or ask an immigrant parent if they go by prevailing folklore and use a poultice of lead-containing earth on an infant's soft spot when it is sunken from dehydration. For families living near an abandoned lead mine and smelter, questions may pertain to whether or not the children play in and eat dirt from that area. Even such rare exposures as the making of leaded windows should not be overlooked. Length of exposure as well as frequency should be determined in order to assess significance.

I (RC) am afraid, though, that by paying so much attention to irrelevant exposure, we have gone overboard. We get exercised about small amounts of lead on completely inedible toys; toys designed for a child far beyond the teething and indiscriminant swallowing age. If such activity is observed, the child should be checked out for having a compulsive disorder or suffering from pica (eating inedible substances) In my state, we used grant money to map out houses built before the ban on indoor lead paint and began blood testing. Houses were mapped for the entire state, with no thought given of the occupants and no knowledge of the child's lead exposure history. Some eight to ten results were over the 10 mcg/dL level. Then, the question had to be asked: What is to be done with these asymptomatic children that were discovered?

Unfortunately, acceptable threshold levels of lead have varied greatly due to an attempt to correlate behavior disorders that are vague, and of multiple etiologies, with lead levels. Many still accept the 10 mcg/dL level as adequate, while others plead for a 5 mcg/dL standard. Some say we should have *no* tolerance for lead, as they claim effects such as a reduction in IQ of one or two points. There have been many attempts to equate very low blood levels with such intangibles as reading disabilities or to equate high-school absenteeism with lead found in deciduous teeth. Even Dr. Needleman, an authority on lead toxicity, who has seen the ups and downs of the standards for lead thresholds to prevent school problems or to determine at what levels to do therapy, admits that he cannot depend completely on laboratory results.

Nutritional deficiencies are a large part of the lead problem. After correcting the deficiencies with good diet and supplementation, and maintaining years of good nutrition, lead simply packs up and leaves. For kids in older houses and apartment buildings, I would suggest checking for anemia; extra iron may need to be prescribed. I would also recommend that children take extra vitamin C. After two months, check to see if the anemia is being corrected.

Mercury

Mercury has been used throughout history. The metal has been found in ancient Egyptian tombs dating back to 1500 B.C. We know that the ancient Chinese found many medicinal uses for mercury. American doctors of the nineteenth century used a mercury compound, Calomel, first as an emetic (bringing about vomiting), then as a laxative. Unfortunately, Calomel became an ingredient of teething powders and found use as an antiseptic. A serious disease called acrodynia, affecting infants, was attributed to the use of calomel teething powders. It is a very dramatic disease with rash, painful and swollen extremities, nervous system disorders, and kidney disease—all of which adds up to producing a very miserable baby.

There are three basic forms of mercury: elemental (inorganic mercury), organic mercury, and salts of mercury. Mercury salts products have mostly been phased out because of safety concerns. Since they do not affect the nervous system, they are considered to be less significant. However, all forms are poisonous if the concentration is high enough over a long enough time.

Inorganic mercury enters our environment by relatively subtle means. Minimata Bay, Japan, was the locus of the most hideous example of industrial pollution and of the "do nothing" attitude of a government authority charged with looking out for the safety of its citizens. In 1956, many cases of infantile cerebral palsy (spastic cerebral palsy) were discovered. It is hard to understand, after witnessing just one of these children with a terribly distorted body, that a search for the cause wasn't undertaken as soon as it was noted that this locale had a much higher incidence of this devastating disorder. Eventually, it became apparent that the culprit was methyl mercury derived from the discharge of a chemical plant. This had been going on with impunity since 1932. Even if some of the pollutant were in the elemental form, it could be converted to the organic form by bacterial action. Shrimp and fish, which made up a big part of the local diet, feasted on lesser organisms that incorporated methyl mercury into their systems. In this way, up the food chain, mercury was eventually passed on to pregnant women and was clearly the cause of the cerebral palsy. The problem was recognized and immediately corrected, right? No! The poisonous discharge continued until 1968.

Methyl mercury is fat-soluble and is well absorbed from the intestinal tract into the bloodstream. It easily enters the placenta and can become part of breast milk. As we have seen with lead toxicity, fetal and infant central nervous system tissues are most vulnerable to damage from this pollutant. One description speaks of methyl mercury "scrambling" the brain. As concentrations increase in the nervous system with long-term exposure, as in adults, symptoms become more severe. Symptoms run the gamut from mild to traumatic—from insomnia, forgetfulness, loss of appetite, mild tremor, stronger tremor, red palms, memory impairment, and excess sweating and salivating, to hearing and visual impairment, spasticity, coma, and death. Early signs and symptoms should be a red flag indicating the need to find the source of pollution, avoid it, and see what can be done about it.

Mercury poisons by binding to sulfur in sulfur-containing amino acids. Some sulfur-containing enzymes essential for life, such as lipoic acid, can be made ineffective from this binding effect. The reaction can be modified with selenium, which stimulates selenium glutathione peroxidase, a powerful antioxidant involved in fat metabolism. Optimal doses of vitamin C are required, not only for its antioxidant effect but also for its chelating action.

Methyl mercury is sometimes used as a fungicide for seed grains. One conscientious mother, to whom I had enthused about the nutritional value of unsalted sunflower seeds, informed me of a surprising finding. She had gone to a "seed and feed store" and asked for some natural sunflower seeds to use for the family. At home, she became concerned about a bluish tint to the seeds. Before feeding them to her children, she let me examine them. I was shocked to find that these seeds had been treated with methyl mercury and that the store personnel had told her they were perfectly suitable for human consumption.

And then there is ethyl mercury. Merthiolate was registered in 1929 as an antiseptic and preservative, and it was once commonly used on scrapes and cuts. Its safety has always been questioned, but no real testing has been done since it was determined "safe" in 1930. Ethyl mercury makes up half of its content. More recently, it has metamorphosed into thimerosal, widely used as a preservative in vaccines. Thimerosal is controversial[10] because many associate the recent rise in autism cases with the use of thimerosal-containing vaccines. The vaccine industry's stance is that this association hasn't been proven. Unfortunately, the scientific papers submitted to the U.S. Food and Drug Administration are either directly from the vaccine manufacturers or from authors who agree with their stance. The other side cannot present a convincing argument without test studies or doing the impossible thing of considering thimerosal the *only* cause of autism. Because some infants who receive thimerosal-containing vaccines might be exposed to more mercury than federal guidelines suggest, the U.S. government asked manufacturers in 1999 to eliminate or reduce the mercury content of their vaccines.[11] Infants are subjected to many more vaccines now than in 1999, so the cumulative effect of mercury should be considered more than ever.

When elemental mercury is volatilized, it is harmful; when in its solid state, it is relatively harmless, with only 0.1 percent absorbed from the gastrointestinal tract. Throwing all forms of mercury into one bad pot can generate a tendency for overkill. Fear of mercury poisoning from a broken thermometer, oral or rectal, is unfounded. The same is true of a broken mercury switch. Mercury dust from a broken fluorescent light is another matter, since the dust can be inhaled like mercury vapor. If breathed in high concentrations, it can

AMALGAM DENTAL FILLINGS

Amalgam is a conglomeration of several metals, predominately mercury (about 50 percent). It was in use in 1845 when a dentist proclaimed that it was "the most objectionable material for filling teeth that can be employed" because of mercury poisoning. It was doubly bad for the dentists of the day because they made their own amalgams. Some dentists were suspended from their dental society for continuing to use amalgam fillings. The American Dental Association (ADA), formed in 1859, changed all that by declaring amalgams safe. They stated that their tests showed that not a significant amount of mercury vapor was released from amalgam fillings. Mercury amalgam was widely used during the Civil War. As early as 1895, it was known that amalgams *did* release significant amounts of mercury vapor. This controversy has now continued for over a hundred years.

There are many studies relating several diseases to a mouthful of amalgams: Alzheimer's disease, fibromyalgia, and some autoimmune diseases. Proof is hard to come by for these diseases of obscure etiology. There are many reports of individuals suffering with one of these problems, then doing better after their amalgams are removed. Of course, "doing better" is a subjective description.

According to the U.S. Consumer Product Safety Commission (CPSC), parents should see that children "avoid fish with high levels of mercury." The CPSC also states, "Keep children and mercury apart: replace mercury thermometers with digital ones. Don't let kids handle or play with mercury."[12] Even though CPSC has information on 4,000 product recalls, there is not a word about dental mercury amalgam fillings. However, in 1995, the CPSC announced a recall of necklaces with small vials or glass balls containing mercury because exposure to their vapor, if they broke, could cause long-term health problems, especially for small children and pregnant women. And one did: a vial broke in a public school in Washington state, which required evacuation of the students until the spill could be cleaned up. It is interesting that the government lets this same toxic metal, in similar quantities, be implanted into kids' living teeth.[13]

Common sense notwithstanding, a panel from the U.S. Food and Drug Administration (FDA) investigating the pros and cons of amalgams, recently released a statement that they found no flaws in their 2009 findings that "dental amalgam fillings are safe for adults and children six years and older." However, they will consider adding a product warning because of "possible health risks that the filling material poses to pregnant women and their fetuses and to young children, particularly nursing mothers."[14] Even if the FDA actually revises the product label, will the dental profession own up to the warning and will patients know anything about it? The ADA praised the study, while a pediatric neurologist said that there is "no place for mercury in children."[15] Sweden, Norway, and Denmark have already banned the use of amalgam dental fillings.[16] Do these countries lack discernment or are they not encumbered by FDA studies?

The FDA's emphasis going forward will be on finding what exactly are "acceptable" levels of mercury vapor that can be released from dental amalgams. Currently, they are referring to standards from the Environmental Protection Agency, but it is much easier to monitor smokestack emissions of mercury than emissions inside the human mouth. No studies measuring the frequency and the forcefulness of "chews" in relationship to release of mercury vapor from amalgam-filled teeth have come to my attention. I have an idea that monitoring instruments in the mouth of a child with bruxism (teeth gnashing) would produce wildly fluctuating recordings.

It is generally accepted that mercury vapor is dangerous when it enters the respiratory system. Fetal, infantile, and young children's nervous systems are particularly vulnerable to damage from mercury. Amalgam fillings do emit mercury vapor that can be inhaled. It is time to think more about the health of infants and children than about arriving at the exact allowable mercury concentration in the human mouth—a concentration that could vary from chew to chew.

The precautionary principle is the simplest and best policy: avoid amalgam fillings. This is easy to do, since mercury-free white composite fillings are readily available. Composite fillings cost slightly more, but they look better cosmetically. Composites are also very durable. Amalgam metal fillings are inserted under pressure and mechanically fill the cavity. Composites are bonded to the tooth, providing a more thorough seal against new decay.

destroy the respiratory tree, causing necrotizing bronchitis and pneumonia. Like inorganic mercury, long-term effects are mainly on the nervous system, but kidney damage can also occur. As with lead poisoning, both the concentration and the length of time of exposure are important factors.

The largest source of mercury in the environment, oddly enough, is from burning coal. Electric power generating in this country comes mainly from coal-fired plants, gas-fired plants, or hydroelectric plants. Mercury content, greater in the organic portion of so-called soft coals, is partially removed by the same "cleaning" processes that remove sulfur. Still, tons of mercury are released into the air every day. China's mercury contribution to a polluted atmosphere can sometimes be detected inland from west coast of the United States.

Mercury rains down from the atmosphere in sufficient quantity to enter into aquatic plants and into the food chain. Couple this with poorly controlled industrial waste and we have a problem with both freshwater bodies and our seas. It is this "unseen enemy" that is hard to defeat. It won't be easy to switch to cleaner forms of electricity generation or to convince the owners of coal-fired plants to invest in more "scrubbers," so our children will not be able to entirely escape mercury exposure. We must protect them with vitamin and trace mineral supplementation.

Little fish on a mercury-contaminated veggie diet are eaten by bigger fish, and on up the chain to the really big fish. Growing up, one of my favorite foods was swordfish steak, but I now know that it was relatively loaded with mercury. Big tuna, swordfish, and shark are listed as the worst offenders of ocean fish. Ironically, many varieties of freshwater fish, desirable for healthy eating because of their omega-3 essential fatty acids, have become contaminated from mercury. It is a difficult to determine how much of these fish can safely be eaten by a pregnant woman or a child in order to get as much of the good fish oil as possible. Concentrations of mercury in the fish have to be figured into the equation. I would like to see studies done that determine mercury levels in salmon, natural (wild) versus farmed, along with omega-3 levels. I suspect that wild salmon, feeding on algae, have a much higher mercury content than farm-raised salmon, which are often fed grains.

Vitamin Supplements Help Protect Children from Heavy Metals

The ability of vitamin C to protect animals from heavy metals is well established. Recent controlled trials with yeast, fish, mice, rats, chickens, clams, guinea pigs, and turkeys all came to the same conclusion: vitamin C protects growing animals from heavy metals poisoning.[17] Benefits with an animal model do not always translate to equal benefits for humans. In this case, however, the benefit has been proven for a wide range of animals, so the odds that vitamin C will protect human children are high.

There is a virtual epidemic of behavior problems, learning disabilities, attention deficit, and autism, and the number of children receiving special education services continues to rise steeply. Although not all causes are yet identified, growing evidence suggests that heavy metal pollution is a significant factor, and vitamin C is part of the solution.

Dr. Erik Paterson, of British Columbia, reports: "When I was a consulting physician for a center for the mentally challenged, a patient showing behavioral changes was found to have blood lead some ten times higher than the acceptable levels. I administered vitamin C at a dose of 4,000 mg/day. I anticipated a slow response. The following year I rechecked his blood lead level. It had gone up, much to my initial dismay. But then I thought that perhaps what was happening was that the vitamin C was mobilizing the lead from his tissues. So we persisted.

The next year, on rechecking, the lead levels had markedly dropped to well below the initial result. As the years went by, the levels became almost undetectable, and his behavior was markedly improved."[18]

Worldwide, coal and high-sulfur fuel oil combustion release close to 300,000 tons of heavy metals annually, a third of which are considered hazardous air pollutants by the U.S. Environmental Protection Agency.[19] This includes arsenic, beryllium, cadmium, cobalt, chromium, mercury, manganese, nickel, lead, antimony, selenium, uranium, and thorium. These metals are also released to the air by the industrial processes that mine and refine metal-containing ores. Heavy metals dispersed into the air as invisible particles are blown by the winds and therefore become widely dispersed.

University of Victoria professor Harold Foster, Ph.D., says, "Pregnant women need special protection because their fetus may be poisoned in the womb, so interfering with its development. In addition to vitamin C, nutrient minerals are also protective against heavy metal toxins. For example, selenium is antagonistic to (and so protective against) arsenic, mercury, and cadmium."[20]

Metals have always been a part of the environment, and our bodies have evolved methods to protect against them. This process involves vitamin-dependent metabolic pathways.[21] Additional vitamin intake, through the use of nutrient supplementation, can help speed up the removal process. Daily consumption of additional vitamin C and selenium is likely to protect children by helping to eliminate heavy metals from their bodies. One easy and inexpensive way to increase intake of these nutrients is by taking a vitamin C supplement with each meal, along with a daily multivitamin containing selenium. Vitamin supplements are remarkably safe for children.[22]

BISPHENOL-A (BPA)

Bisphenol-A (BPA) is a polluting chemical that we can, and must, do something about. It is used to make the polycarbonate plastic found in clear, hard plastic containers. Since the mid-1930s, BPA has been known to have estrogen-like properties. Not until the present have steps been taken to protect fetuses, infants, and children, the usual target population that the FDA *finally* identifies. Ironically, because of BPA's use as a liner of cans (including infant formula cans) and the substance of baby bottles, infants can receive high exposure. Heating formula in one of these bottles produces leaching of the chemical and higher levels in babies. As usual, the FDA staunchly defends its safety standards for this chemical, while independent studies report levels in humans that are sometimes ten times higher than this standard. (The FDA states: "Infant formula, including infant formula packaged in cans, is a safe and acceptable alternative. . . . [The] FDA is not recommending that families change the use of infant formula or foods, as the benefit of a stable source of good nutrition outweighs the potential risk of BPA exposure."[23])

In concern for our target population, children show higher levels than adolescents do, who show higher levels than adults do. We have to remember that the fetus and infant are the most vulnerable of all. Japan banned BPA use in baby bottles in 1997; Canada and the European Union have followed suit. Public pressure will probably cause the FDA to have a change of heart in the near future, and some formula producers have voluntarily switched to a safer can liner. Why is the FDA fifteen years behind the times?

The endocrine-disrupting property of BPA has been known and studied for decades. BPA disturbs thyroid metabolism as well as disrupting dopaminergic systems (factors involved in Parkinson's disease and neurotransmitter formation). Most serious is the estrogen effect, since it goes into action in the early life of the fetus. One study relates the association of early fetal exposure in females with a masculinizing effect that creates aggressiveness in older girls.[24] Studies involving soy phytoestrogens, organophosphate pesticides, and other proven or suspected estrogen look-alikes show an association of these hormone disrupters with abnormalities in raising male genitalia: microphallus (small penis), an undescended or absent testicle, or smaller testicles in young adults. The counterpart in females is shown in the much earlier onset of puberty in girls and earlier onset of menopause in women, explained by too much stimulation of ovaries, or burning out, from surrogate estrogens.

Even though the FDA is slow to respond to the overwhelming evidence of toxicity due to BPA, other countries have banned its use for baby bottles. Manufacturers of baby bottles have voluntarily switched to other materials. There are seven different kinds of plastic, some of which contain BPA. In general, check out all plastic food or liquid containers and never heat substances in the suspected ones. BPA is not likely to leach out from a cold container.

DES

Like a meteor streaking across the sky, diethylstilbestrol (DES), an estrogen derivative, had a flashy but short life on the medical scene. It was felt that it would reduce the incidence of pregnancy complications, including miscarriages. Its life was terminated when it was found to be the cause of a rare type of vaginal tumor in girls and young women who had been exposed to DES in the womb. We don't have to worry about avoiding DES, because it was taken off the market around 1970. I include it due to the revelations that it may cause a higher incidence of reproductive disorders than expected in both girls and boys in the second generation. (When the affected female fetus grew up and had children of her own, the problem was passed on to the next generation.) Some studies suggest that similar problems were passed on to the third generation.[25] This unacceptable outcome from a hormone that could be passed down to future generations prompted a closer look at other hormone disrupters. In doing so, I found research indicating feminization of some male animals, showing that not only DES but other endocrine disrupters cause structural neurological changes.[26] These changes were associated with gender-related behavioral changes.

We don't have the space in this chapter to touch on all the household products, cosmetics, and skin care products that *might* be toxic. We not only can't get beyond the "might," but our government agencies are way behind in establishing safety levels of chemicals that have been on the market for decades, let alone the myriad of new products constantly entering the market. We are in an environmental toxic soup. Avoid the obvious, don't sweat the little stuff, and by all means eat well and take your vitamins.

FLUORIDATION

I am solidly against fluoride supplementation, because I think the "science" of fluoridation is basically badly flawed. Fluoride supplementation is made the key to dental health, many times to the exclusion of other nutritional contributions.

Ever since the association was made between fewer dental caries and a certain range of fluoride concentration in community drinking water, organized health establishments, one by one, fell in line by recommending fluoridation of public water supplies. Immediately, those of us who opposed this action were made to feel we were subversive types who liked neither nice teeth nor their owners.

The basic tenet of fluoridation is one I have never been able to swallow: don't be concerned about absolute amounts of ingested fluoride, only the concentration. Why medically trained people accept this is beyond me. Can you imagine dispensing a drug such as digitalis as a standard concentration, in drop form, based on an average adult weight and instructing the patient to take precisely so many drops daily, either all at once or spread throughout the day in increments that will equal the prescribed total dose? The gold standard for fluoridating water is 1 mg per liter. Neither the size of the person nor the volume of water consumed enter into the equation, as if every creature, big or small, in weather that is either hot or cold, has the same need. Are a twenty-pound infant and a fourteen-year-old boy out for late summer football practice going to require or imbibe the same amount of fluoridated water?

I know enough about the source of fluoride for fluoridation purposes to be skeptical. Fluorine, which is toxic to plants, is driven out of rock phosphate by heat and acid as it is converted into water-soluble phosphate fertilizer. If it goes out the smoke stack, it causes foliage denuding in the surrounding area. Years ago, at the plant at Garrison, Montana, adjacent to our natural fertilizer plant in which we merely ground the rock phosphate, it caused crippling brittle bone disease in cattle. Releasing fluoride from bauxite at the Columbia Falls, Montana, aluminum plant similarly denuded the surrounding hills. If the fluorine is captured in fertilizer production, the question is what do we do with this substance. This was a substantial problem for the fertilizer industry until public health officials found an acceptable dumping ground for it—public drinking water supplies. Substantiating evidence for fluoride's effect on cavities conveniently came during the "energy crisis," when fertilizer demand and production were down, and some fluoridated communities could not get fluoride for their water supply.

I am skeptical of any health program that is costly, particularly if it requires expensive equipment. City governing bodies have been subjected to a lot of pressure by pro-fluoridationists, who attempt to promote their program with claims that the metering instrumentation is flawless, that there will be no added costs of maintenance of water distribution lines, that there are no health drawbacks such as mottling of the enamel of children's teeth or sensitivity reactions, and that studies have shown that there is a 40–60 percent reduction in the incidence of dental caries. Of course, no machines can be guaranteed to perform flawlessly, nor can their operators.

Arguments for fluoridation are surprisingly weak. *Infant Nutrition*[28] by Samuel J. Forman, a professor of pediatrics at the University of Iowa Medical School, was long considered the bible of pediatric nutrition. In the 1974 edition, the book proposes several theories on fluoride and cavities:

1. Some of the calcium phosphate in teeth (and bone) takes up trace amounts of fluoride to form calcium fluorapatite, a complex crystal similar to the compound we call rock phosphate. It is extremely resistant to attack by acids. But Dr. Forman diminishes the importance of this, apparently because fluorapatite is in such small amounts in normal tooth enamel, making the overall enamel only a bit more acid resistant.

2. In exceedingly small amounts, fluoride enhances the rate of remineralization of enamel.

3. Fluoride suppresses the metabolic activities of decay-causing (cariogenic) bacteria in the mouth. Higher concentrations of fluoride, which occur when fluoride is applied directly to the tooth surface,

or when a child sucks on a fluoride tablet, reduce the concentration of *Streptococcus mutans* in the dental plaque. I always thought this must be the way it is effective; it is simply an antiseptic in higher concentrations.

4. Fluoride interferes with the ability of microorganisms to form plaque. This is similar to the process previously mentioned, or the two may be considered to be on a continuum, both acting topically rather than systemically. But if fluoride acts topically, why put it in water?

I find it interesting that proponents of fluoride supplementation strive to appear so "scientific" about the optimal amounts and times of ingestion, yet all of the above explanations of the action of fluoride are called *possible* mechanisms. The systemic benefit might come into play here from swallowing the topical application, but precise amounts cannot possibly be determined.

Every few years, the American Academy of Pediatrics (AAP) publishes a *Pediatric Nutrition Handbook*. In the 1979 edition, they speak of safe levels of prescribed fluoride based on whether mottling of the enamel is produced. They admit that there is mottling but that

FLUORIDE: THE BEGINNING OF THE END?

The U.S Centers for Disease Control and Prevention (CDC) recently reduced the recommended fluoride concentration in public water supplies from 1 ppm (parts per million) to 0.7 ppm. Strangely (finally), the CDC now is saying that over half of U.S. children are overexposed to fluoride, especially infants on either liquid or powdered formulas mixed with fluoridated water. While difficult to do with water intake, we need to adjust the amount of fluoride according to size, ambient temperature, and activity. Since this is impractical, overdose is likely. Therefore, at least for your children, avoid fluoridated water. If this is hard to do, have pure water displace some of the fluoridated tap water.

it may be at an acceptable level. Now, the mottling I have seen consists of very noticeable chalky white spots in the permanent incisors (the middle of the smile), which start to form their enamel at 3–4 months of age, with the process completed by 4–5 years of age. Since there is no known etiology for these characteristic spots other than fluoride ingestion, we must grant that this deformity represents fluoride toxicity, at least for that individual. Perhaps, as with vitamins, there is variation in individual needs. And perhaps a dentist who is a loyal fluoride fan can more easily accept mottling than the child's mother. The more flagrant cases of fluorosis are readily noted because the spots are brown.

So, we have two modes of usefulness of fluoride that are presented, systemic and topical. If one were to attempt to promote both modes, watch out for negating arguments. Those promoting fluoridating water supplies seem to feel that the main value is to ingest fluoridated water during enamel development; since a once-a-day form of supplement (one slug) is rapidly excreted by the kidneys, getting a dash of fluoride several times a day through the water is better. Do the small increments of fluoride enhance the remineralization of the enamel or work topically, perhaps to do in those nasty cariogenic bacteria?

Those promoting prescribed daily fluoride supplements must also reckon with many arguments. In the AAP handbook, fluoride is not mentioned under "trace minerals," which it is (like copper, zinc, magnesium, and so on). They recommend a downward adjustment of the fluoride supplemental dose from their previous recommendation. Supplementation is felt to be the second best way of providing fluoride, since "health authorities agree that, in communities where the fluoride concentration of the water is suboptimal, the most effective and inexpensive means of reducing dental decay is by adjusting the community water supply to an optimal fluoride concentration." I am certain that all health authorities do *not* agree.

The biggest drawback to fluoride drops is mottling. The development of mottling from ingesting too much fluoride is not as much of a problem in early infancy, but after six months of age, fluoride intake must be carefully assessed. The goal of the AAP is to find out the fluoride concentration of the drinking water of each patient and add enough supplement to make a total daily intake of the magical 1 mg. Here's where things get complicated:

- In communities with a fluoride concentration of less than 0.5 ppm or 0.5 mg/liter, give 0.5 mg from birth to three years of age; 1 mg for those over three years.

- If the water supply was greater than 0.5 ppm, no supplementation is needed.

- In communities with less than 0.2 ppm fluoride in the water supply, the recommendation is 0.25 mg of fluoride daily between birth and two years of age; 0.5 mg between two and three years; 1 mg after age three.

The upshot of all this is the necessity for a physician to know the fluoride concentration of his or her patients' drinking water and write a prescription for the appropriate strength of fluoride drops to constitute a total appropriate dose for three different age groups. The physician is not to "complicate" the issue with questions of individual differences of ingestion or weight.

> *Dental fluorosis (tooth mottling) is now estimated at 41 percent among adolescents aged 12–15 in the United States.*[27]

Infant foods and beverages also contain fluoride in previously unsuspected amounts, and there is the admission that we don't know the quantity of fluoride toothpaste that children swallow. The revised 1985 AAP handbook has some interesting thoughts to ponder: "Because these sources of fluoride are so variable, they cannot be reliably estimated for any patient. Neither can water consumption, which can vary tremendously from one child to another. However, the fluoride concentration of a patient's water supply is accepted as the best indicator of dietary exposure to fluoride." These sensible arguments are negated by this: "The optimal intake of fluoride from all sources is estimated to be 0.05 mg fluoride per kilogram body weight per day.

Obviously, a supplementation regime based on body weight would be the most desirable, although it is also the most complicated. Therefore, the dosage regime is geared to the patient's age for simplicity."[29] My feeling is, if you can't do it right, don't do it at all. To further add to problems of compliance, it is pointed out that sodium fluoride should be given between meals or at bedtime so that calcium-rich foods will not interfere with absorption.

Other Options for Good Dental Health

I (RC) say, forget about precisely prescribed fluoride supplementation. We know very little about the interrelationships between fluoride and other nutrients, and the exact amounts an individual needs. More attention should be placed on how we achieve good dental health by having a healthy dentin throughout the formation of teeth and learning proper nutrition, which would provide better health for other cells of the body as well. Besides the usual dental hygiene measures, such as brushing and flossing (for the older child), fluoride emphasis has preempted other strategies to reduce the incidence of cavities. Dental health education should include means of getting substrates of plaque formation off of the teeth as soon as possible after eating sugars and starchy foods by cleaning the tongue, swishing water in the mouth, eating a cleansing food, or brushing. Baking soda and some factor in aged cheese have been shown to have anticariogenic effects, presumably from their action on the oral flora. Certainly, these substances are much less toxic than fluoride. Foods that require chewing, rather than concentrated calories that slide down easily, promote better gum health as well as increasing saliva production, which is anticariogenic. Certainly, nutrition that promotes good health for the teeth themselves is also promoting good health for the supporting tissues—gingivae and periodontal bone. These things must be considered for adult dental health, since fluoride intake has little impact on periodontal disease.

I think these various health advisory committees have painted themselves into a corner by strongly advocating fluoridation of water supplies or supplementing daily doses before contrary evidence was aired. Still, in some circles, an opinion in opposition to fluoridation or fluoride supplementation is regarded as uninformed if not downright un-American. On the other hand, maybe opposition is warranted. Dental fluorosis (discoloration and mottling of the teeth) is now officially estimated to affect 41 percent of all adolescents ages 12–15 in the U.S.[30]

SUMMARY

With environmental pollutants, the only way to win is not to play. Avoid as many known toxic chemicals as you possibly can. Read labels and keep up-to-date at the library and on the Internet. Buy organic if you can afford to; start your own organic garden if you cannot. If you cannot do either, wash any produce that lends itself to washing just like you wash your hands: with soap and water, followed by rinsing. Common dishwashing detergents or soap will remove much, probably most, pesticide residues. Our general rule with chemicals: simply leave them out.

Think outside of the dental chair. Good diet helps prevents cavities. Always choose white composite fillings, since they are mercury free. Rethink fluoride: some may be good, but kids are getting far too much.

OBESITY AND DIABETES

PART THREE

MAJOR
CHILDREN'S
HEALTH
PROBLEMS

CHAPTER 8

OBESITY AND DIABETES

"Disease is the censor pointing out the humans,
animals and plants who are imperfectly nourished."
—G.T. WRENCH, *THE WHEEL OF HEALTH*

Childhood obesity is receiving a lot of attention and will continue to, and justly so. In 2008, figures from the National Center for Chronic Disease Prevention and Health Promotion showed a tripling of childhood obesity in the United States in the past thirty years:

- In those six to eleven years old, from 6.5 percent to 19.6 percent

- In those twelve to nineteen years old, from 5 percent to 18.1 percent

Other sources are in agreement, but some present even higher rates of increase. Even worse, the figure for the incidence of overweight adults in the U.S. may be over 60 percent. It appears that there has been an exponential rate of increase in just the last decade.

THE CULTURE OF OBESITY

First, let us look at the cultural changes over the past thirty years that have accompanied this emerging health crisis. As we do, we can see many concerned people working hard to bring back healthy patterns that used to keep obesity in check but have been neglected during this period.

Organized school sports are a given, but they are entering the lives of children at a progressively earlier age. This is fine for the majority of participants but puts the overweight kid on the fringe. Regular physical education that encourages participation by all has often been entirely dropped from the school curriculum or reduced from being an everyday event to only once a week. Less attention has been paid to healthy meal preparation or to what comes out of school cafeterias for school lunches.

The amazing thing is how obesity in children has been overlooked. We have all heard of the frog (but has anyone seen it?) that was put in a pot of water on the stove. The heat of the water slowly, but surely, increased until the frog, without protest, was boiled. Is weight gain so subtle that we can't see it? Why don't we hop out of the pot? We can if we really want to—if we understand the seriousness of obesity or if we believe and act on what we constantly hear concerning healthy diets and the necessity of exercise. I am sorry to see less emphasis on the well-child check-up. A health professional can tactfully point out what the parent has not readily seen. In the beginning of a trend of weight gain, there is not the "sensitivity" issue to deal with, and corrective measures are more readily accepted.

The childhood obesity problem has sneaked up on the nation due to neglect (and lack of emphasis on "well" checks) from doctors and parents alike. Children's adult role models have also been caught in obesity's web. Obese people are neither ignorant nor stubborn. They are among those affected by a general attitude of "everybody's doing it, I'm doing fine, and I see no dire consequences coming from the way I live." If disaster hasn't yet struck the adult, it seems unlikely to affect a healthy (appearing) youngster. There is so much "noise" about unhealthy diets and so few specifics of what constitutes a healthy diet for the individual. Being bombarded with health information that seems so general reaches the point of diminishing returns—much like the boy who cried "wolf." Even when one accepts new ways of feeding the family, it requires major steps to learn how to shop for "real" food that is healthy *and* affordable. In many neighborhoods, outlets for fresh produce and unprocessed foods are scarce or nonexistent.

A REALLY HEALTHY ROLE MODEL: JACK LALANNE

Even before I (AWS) was of school age, I recall that when my mother took off her kitchen apron and started pushing the dinette chairs out of the way, it was time for the Jack LaLanne Show. Of course, she had to turn on our ancient TV a good five minutes ahead of time, to let it warm up. I usually stuck around for the program, mostly as an excuse to see LaLanne's big white German Shepherd dog, Happy. But my line of work today shows just what a strong, if subliminal, impression the incredibly cheerful, incredibly agile Mr. LaLanne had made on me.

Rising every morning at 5 AM, Jack LaLanne stayed both agile and cheerful. He did a two-hour workout every single day, saying, "You don't get old from age; you get old from inactivity." That's a good point. A survey of persons over 100 years of age found that the one thing almost all centenarians have in common is that they have something that they absolutely, positively must do tomorrow.

And Mr. LaLanne said: "The only way you can hurt this body is "don't do it." Sit around on your big, fat behind and think of the good old days, or make some excuse why you're not doing it."

People have always called enthusiasts like Jack LaLanne "health nuts." Well, what other kind of nut would you want to be? A disease nut?

Said Mr. LaLanne in a TV interview: "I was into juicing. And you know, I was a nut. I was a filbert! I was a crackpot. That just shows you, right? You see, my life was saved. I was a skinny, weak, miserable, sugar-holic kid. At age 15, I attended a health lecture, and I quit eating meat, and I ate natural foods, and I started exercising. My whole life changed. If something changed your life, wouldn't you be enthusiastic about it?"[1]

And in *USA Today,* he said:

"I have only two rules for eating well: If man made it, don't eat it. That includes synthetic sweeteners and food dyes. And keep everything in natural balance. This means eating whole grain cereals rather than overly processed ones, and eating fresh fruit and vegetables instead of canned ones, or those sweetened with processed sugars."[2]

LaLanne entered the health business in 1936. His TV shows ran for 34 years, a Guinness World Record. He is a chiropractic college graduate. He received his own star on the Hollywood Walk of Fame.[3]

He was quite a man, way ahead of his time: a self-described "sugar kid" who turned to good nutrition and exercise. Many people are aware of his advocacy for raw fruit and vegetable juices. But his brilliance was in demonstrating his exercises, in which he used no complicated apparatus, usually just a towel and a chair. He encouraged everyone to work out at a time when there was fear that exercise made you "muscle bound." He said, "Exercise is your King; nutrition is your Queen. Together they are your Kingdom." He influenced our thinking about fresh vegetable juices, because here was a guy that gave an incredible example by doing what he believed. "I can't die," Jack often said. "It would ruin my image!" He coined a good phrase, but he made it to age 96. There is a moral in here somewhere. If a 90-plus year old gentleman can be a "filbert" and get up every morning and exercise, well, darn it, so can we. At any age, and the sooner the better.

We realize that being grossly overweight in any age group is fraught with questions of self-esteem and being able to fit in. However, dwelling on a "poor me" attitude provides a disincentive to take positive, corrective steps. This faulty attitude can feed a sense of inevitability, hopelessness, and isolation. Shouldn't we be making more of an effort before allowing the drastic step of childhood gastric bypass surgery? Looking at one's self realistically, with the help of friends, family, and teachers, gets one on a corrective path. For it will take all the support possible to disavow a sense of hopelessness and begin a positive program. A better way to achieve self-esteem is to truly deserve it, to have the gumption to say, "My present state is no longer acceptable. I'll get off my tail and burn some calories. I'll listen to those who can instruct me about good nutrition and develop the discipline to try, then adopt, new tastes."

For the child, substituting outdoor physical activity for playing indoors with an electronic gadget pays other dividends. Peers respect seeing the attempts at taking hold of the problem rather than further withdrawing from contact with them. Eventually, physical fitness improvement, with a gain in athletic prowess, can help boys or girls gain entrance into team sports and the creation of real friendships. Children, like their adult counterparts, quickly understand the association of physical health with mental health. Positive attitude and the improvement of energy level go hand in hand. The trick is in biting the bullet and making a start. As the program progresses, one appreciates how feeling better also means feeling good about one's self.

Unfortunately, bullying is a persistent problem in schools. A noticeably overweight kid is inevitably going to be taunted with the "fat" word, not "overweight" or "obese." Depending on the type of support at home, a child victim can go into a funk or be encouraged to take an honest look at the situation. Certainly, the tormentors are dead wrong, but the problem with tormentors is that they won't fade away. An obvious rhetorical question would be, "Why do you suppose they said you were fat?" With loving support and understanding, the taunts could be motivating.

Neither doctors nor parents need charts to tell us that a child is overweight. Actually, "overweight" is a non sequitur: an NFL linebacker, all muscle, is overweight (according to his BMI figure), but by no stretch of the imagination is he fat. With just a glance, we can all differentiate fat from muscle. If a person is fat, his or her risk for medical problems down the road is increased dramatically. Doomsayers are pretty grim as they calculate the impact of obesity on healthcare delivery in just a few decades.

So, what excuse do we have for not nipping the problem in the bud? We know that this is a problem of faulty lifestyle, preponderantly from poor nutrition and lack of exercise. Yet, the idea persists that we can find a medical cure, or better, a miraculous "gene" cure.

Since the mapping of the human genome, we have heard the hype about the possibilities of cures for many serious medical problems. There are only a few serious diseases whose outcomes are determined by genes that don't respond to any outside influence. Most genes work in concert with other genes, one regulating the other. We overlook the fact that genes simply determine the blueprint for enzymes that govern our metabolic functions. Enzyme function is largely determined by the levels of vitamin-containing cofactors that are part of coenzymes, without which enzymes do not function. There are many recognized vitamin-deficiency diseases that can be corrected with vitamin therapy. Deficiencies of a degree not severe enough to cause noticeable disease are keeping the enzyme system functioning below an optimal level. On the other hand, enzyme function and regulation can often be increased with the addition of more coenzyme, by supplying more of its vitamin or mineral component. We can hope for gene therapy breakthroughs in the future, but we have nutrition knowledge *now.*

FOOD IS OUR FUEL

Both the factors of *becoming* obese and in *being* obese lead to many serious health problems that, if left unchecked, may progress to the development of type 2 diabetes. The most simple and direct factor in becoming overweight is overeating. Food is our fuel for energy production and body maintenance. If we take in more fuel than we need or can use at the moment, we store up the excess for lean times. So, eat less and burn more with exercise. In addition to paying attention to the amount of fuel, we need to be smart about the type of fuels we ingest, which have different fates in terms of energy production and storage.

The hormone insulin, produced in islands of cells in the pancreas, has a powerful regulatory job. It helps get our food substances either in shape for being utilized for fuel, rebuilding, or storage. It works in conjunction with other hormones in a checks-and-balances fashion.

Early man, as a hunter and gatherer, lived on a feast-or-famine

basis. Insulin enabled humans to meet their immediate energy requirements during feast and store the excess as fat, in fat cells or as glyco-
gen (from carbohydrates) in liver and muscle, in preparation for the
next famine. When under stress from an encounter with a ferocious
beast, adrenaline and other stress hormones were released. These
substances counter insulin's effect and mobilize fat and glucose
(sugar) for enabling the "fight or flight" response. Ideally, just enough
energy-building precursors would be released to satisfy immediate
energy needs. Realistically, there can be an excess that calls on insulin
to go into its storage mode.

The seesaw regulatory system worked very well, and would work
well in modern society, if we could find a way to switch on the stress
hormones only when under extreme circumstances and switch them
off as soon as the crisis is over. In our modern culture, since food fuel
is nearly always available, the storage mechanism is rarely called
upon. Less potent stress-producing situations ("beasts" less ferocious,
such as a traffic jam) found today, even those our children constantly encounter, are not sufficient to trigger the survival response that
would immediately utilize the available fuel. So insulin is called into
play to store the excess.

In addition to stress factors, the type of fuel is of great importance.
We see the fat mingled in with the flesh of the animals we eat is similar to what we call "fat" in our bodies. Also, weight for weight, fat
has over twice the calories of protein or carbohydrate. The focus,
then, has been on reducing consumption of animal fat—or worse, all
fats—in order to combat obesity. It has been hard to let go of this
inadequate, simplistic view but, increasingly, attention is turning to
the *real* culprit, refined carbohydrates. The new thesis can be further
narrowed to the overwhelming intake of high-fructose corn syrup
(HFCS) by children.

A calorie is a calorie, so how could this be? There is more to it
than that. What happens in the body is much more complicated. We
have to gain an understanding of the metabolism of the various types
of carbohydrates and not link them all together—the mistake we
made thinking of fat, not fats.

There is a common pathway for the major food groups (carbohydrate, protein, and fat) in transforming each into substances that either produce energy or become the building blocks for repair and growth. This is called the Krebs cycle or citric acid cycle, the final oxidation (burning) and energy production for all metabolic fuels. It is an electron exchange system that works through vitamin-containing enzymes. The intermediary products can be taken out of the cycle to enter pathways for either more energy production or more building blocks. The whole system is marvelously controlled by enzymes that are activated according to need, behaving like toggle switches controlled by sensors, turning on or off one pathway or the other. The end products down the chains of reactions for each of carbohydrate, protein, and fat are coupled with a coenzyme, which allows entry into the cycle. Since the breakdown products of each of the food groups go into a common pool, individuality is diminished. The focus on fats only, neglecting the fates of carbohydrates and proteins, has impeded progress.

What Happens to Ingested Carbohydrates?

The ultimate carbohydrate metabolic fuel is glucose. In foods, it is found by itself, coupled with another simple sugar (disaccharides, such as sucrose or table sugar), or with many units of glucose joined together to form starch. Enzymes in saliva start the digestive process, and a pancreatic enzyme released into the small intestine completes the conversion to glucose. An early enzymatic step prepares glucose for entry into intestinal cells, then into the bloodstream, on to the liver and the beginning of energy production. This step is stimulated by insulin and the enzyme responsible for the step shuts down when energy needs are met. In the liver, this enzyme function is increased in response to a greater load of glucose following a meal. Many metabolic steps, requiring vitamin-containing enzymes, are taken to gain entry into the Krebs cycle. The first step and third step are rate limiting for glucose but not for fructose, meaning that if energy needs are met, energy production stops at that enzymatic step.

Half of sucrose (table sugar) or the sugar of fruits can go side by side with glucose in the metabolic process unless the common pathway is overrun with fructose. Because fructose escapes the rate-limiting process, in large amounts it overwhelms glucose metabolism. (Some experts in the nutrition field refer to an abnormally large fructose intake as *perturbing* glucose metabolism.) We are designed to be able to include fructose-containing fruit—our gut providing the "limiting" factor—but not the huge amounts of fructose in soda drinks that children might drink. The Center for Science in the Public Interest notes that from 1978 to 1999, soda consumption was three times greater in teenaged boys and two times greater in girls, with some boys drinking as many as five cans or more per day of soda, containing the equivalent of ten teaspoons of sugar.[4] Since then, we have gone from "sugar" (which is one-half fructose) to mostly high-fructose corn syrup, and we have greatly increased the serving size.

Fake sweeteners are no improvement. There are many recent studies coming to the surface about the toxicity of diet soft drinks. We have known about aspartame toxicity for quite some time, and many question why it was ever approved in the first place. Avoid toxic aspartame found in diet pop with total abstinence from such beverages. The other ingredients of diet pop are food dyes and, all too often, caffeine. Kids do not need those.

The Importance of Calcium

Here is the big problem—soda has displaced milk. Calcium deficiency is not likely to be a frequent problem until school age. It is well known that breast milk and cow's milk formulas are both good food sources. Unless the source is not available, or there is an absorption or allergy problem, we should not worry about our normal children until they enter the "pop" age. Sodas can displace milk intake at far too early an age. Many teenagers and young parents may think of milk as being the stuff for little kids and may substitute juice or water for milk if they are convinced that soda is bad.

Adolescence is the time to build bones. The issue of calcium intake is something very important to think about, especially for girls in their teens. This is the time when the good bones of women in their forties and fifties are being predetermined. For a growing child over five years old, recommendations vary from 800–1200 mg of calcium per day.

Dairy products are still a good calcium source, and cultured dairy is especially good. For example, 1.5 ounces of hard cheese provides 300 mg of calcium, the same as 8 ounces of milk or yogurt. Cultured milk products, such as buttermilk and yogurt, have many health advantages. And low-fat yogurt (*low-* not *non-*, since some fat is needed for the good bacteria to feast on) weighs in at 415 mg per 8 ounces (over a third better than plain milk). Another ready source is 300 mg of any common calcium-based (usually calcium carbonate) antacid. If the daily recommendation is not met by the end of the day, take a tablet containing 300 mg after dinner. When the diet is heavy in acid-forming meat and other protein sources and light in alkaline-forming fruits and vegetables, more calcium is used to neutralize urine and lost from the body, leaving less for bone metabolism. Along with adequate vitamin D and exercise, calcium is used more efficiently and not as much is needed.

Other sources do not come up to the level of milk products, but coupled with other lifestyle factors they may prove adequate. These are: sardines (91 mg in two little ones, soft bones and all), sunflower seeds (4 ounces contains 33 mg of calcium but a whopping 100 mg of magnesium, half the daily requirement), and leafy green vegetables (10 ounces of raw spinach contains 202 mg calcium and half a cup of boiled has 139 mg but is relatively heavy in magnesium at 65 mg). Peanuts and dried beans offer much less calcium but are a moderately good source of magnesium. Soybeans deserve a special dispensation in that, depending on how they are prepared, they are relatively abundant in both calcium and magnesium. A half-cup of raw, firm tofu yields 258 mg of calcium and 118 mg of magnesium. A half-cup of dry roasted soybeans yields 232 mg of calcium and 196 mg of magnesium, which meets the daily requirement. Other sources of calcium and magnesium include almonds, whole grains, and figs. (We have given magnesium values at the same time as those for calcium because magnesium is required to aid the metabolism of calcium.)

DIABETES

Diabetes is the failure to metabolize glucose due to insulin lack or inefficiency. Type 1 diabetes is an autoimmune disease in which the body attacks its own insulin-producing cells of the pancreas, so that insulin can no longer be released as needed. Insulin, from that time on, must be given by artificial means (shot or insulin pump), while estimating the proper times for administration depending on testing blood glucose levels and balancing caloric intake with exercise. Symptoms are profound and the disease progresses rapidly. Since glucose is unable to enter the energy-producing pathway, there is hunger. Because there is insufficient insulin to put glucose into storage, the glucose spills over into the urine and demands great quantities of water to go along with it. The brain does not metabolize fat but is instead dependent on glucose, so mental sluggishness results, which can progress to coma if insulin is not administered.

By contrast, type 2 diabetes develops more slowly, depending on the degree of input of all the factors we have discussed. The tug of war between hyperinsulinism and its antagonists results in insulin resistance. Insulin production can be overwhelmed by too heavy a load of glucose, and its ability to stimulate the metabolic process of energy production from glucose is weakened. In turn, it can no longer adequately suppress the action of the hormones that stimulate the making of new glucose. At the same time, higher glucose levels overwhelm muscle insulin receptors, where energy production is needed, but insulin receptors in fat are still able to do their job. The combination of the burnout of insulin from overproduction with the imbalance of insulin receptors means more body fat and less energy. The liver continues to produce more glucose even as it is flooded with glucose, while insulin response to rising glucose levels falls short.

Once the cycle is under way, blood glucose levels will continue to rise unless there is intervention. When blood glucose levels are too high, intervention might include insulin shots. Any blood glucose level that exceeds the normal value should be a cause of great concern that calls for rapid correction.

The Role of Insulin in Diabetes Complications

In Chapter 6, we described what is referred to as "cholesterol" not as "free" cholesterol but as part of lipoprotein complexes, some of which are considered "good" and some "bad." The significance of dietary cholesterol intake pales in comparison to its synthesis in the liver. The initial step of cholesterol synthesis in the liver is controlled by a rate-limiting enzyme, which means that if more cholesterol is not needed, more is not made. Overfeeding of cholesterol actually reduces liver synthesis; however, insulin stimulates liver synthesis. The cholesterol-lowering drugs called statins reduce the activity of the rate-limiting enzyme and attempt to nip cholesterol synthesis in the bud. So, there is a battle between the statins and insulin for control of cholesterol levels. If a person has hyperinsulinism, insulin will probably prove victorious. Also in insulin's favor is its role in raising triglyceride levels, which compose as much as 80 percent of very low-density lipoproteins (VLDLs).

Hyperinsulinism has been shown to lead to the development of artery disease. Of special importance are the coronary arteries that supply oxygen and nutrients to the heart muscle itself. Whether or not cholesterol is the principal culprit in narrowing the lumen (inside space) of the arteries, it is certainly part of the process. When the inner lining of an artery is damaged (perhaps by high blood pressure), repair proceeds normally if vitamin C is present in sufficient amounts. If not, a surrogate (substitute) substance called plasminogen, a precursor of plasmin, takes its place, preventing the formation of a temporary, healing clot. Apolipoprotein(a), an apoprotein that is part of a cholesterol-containing lipoprotein, is also a look-alike of vitamin C and enters into the unhealed area. This plaque-forming cholesterol displaces plasmin, a clot dissolver that breaks down fibrinogen. This process is called plaque buildup and is responsible for artery narrowing, which can starve the heart and other muscles of sufficient oxygen and nutrients.

A high blood glucose level due to inadequate insulin function is, in itself, a health hazard. The formation of free radicals that cause oxidative damage occurs as the body metabolizes food for fuel. Free radicals are highly reactive rogue molecules that damage and age cells. More of these free radicals are formed in proportion to the amount of fuel being metabolized. Plus, glucose is more inclined to undergo auto-oxidation (a process that feeds on itself) than some other metabolic fuels.

If the problems of type 2 diabetes are left unattended, they can evolve into the complications of type 1 diabetes. Whether from free radical damage or as a direct effect on endothelial dysfunction (how the lining of small arteries and capillaries dilate or constrict), high blood levels of glucose cause microvascular disease. Poor control of blood glucose levels can lead to retinal disease, including hemorrhage, which may progress to blindness, or to damage to small blood vessels in the kidney, which can lead to kidney failure. As the lumen of larger arteries becomes progressively narrower—a condition known as peripheral artery disease—can lead to amputation of toes or even higher up the leg. A frequent, but more poorly understood problem, is peripheral neuropathy, usually pain in the feet sometimes described as "walking on tacks." Poor circulation from damaged peripheral arteries, coupled with damaged peripheral nerves, can cause skin ulcers that are difficult to heal.

The only encouraging news about these complications is that they often require years to develop, even without good diabetes management. If fear is ever a good motivation to do something positive, this "doomsday" description should fit the bill.

WHAT YOU CAN DO ABOUT OBESITY AND DIABETES

First of all, don't let it happen. It is easier to prevent excessive weight gain than to lose weight. The gaining process itself initiates many unhealthy patterns that progress if not reversed. If weight gain (with fat accumulating where it shouldn't) sneaks up on your child or other family members, don't deny what you see but get to work. The condition won't go away on its own and requires a disciplined plan of attack. The foundation of prevention or treatment is diet and exercise. Favorable changes require dedication and confidence that the goal of weight loss is within reach.

Exercise

The most difficult part of an exercise program is getting started. If other family members can join in, the task is made easier and demonstrates belief in the benefits. An outdoor activity is best: walking, bicycling, swimming, or whatever the weather and location allow. In inclement weather, consider walking in a nearby protected area like a mall or doing "steps" or aerobic dancing at home.

Take an inventory of your child's activity in order to gauge the starting point. If your child has been downright sedentary, simply moving will represent a start. Make it clear that the exercise program is a progressive program with realistic, achievable goals. It will be hard at first, but gains in strength, positive attitude, and just feeling better come early on and provide reinforcement. Patience and discipline are required. This is not a "quick fix" program but rather a long-term—even lifelong—program. Exercise produces more insulin receptors in muscle, where glucose is utilized for energy production rather than entering the pathway toward fat storage, which is activated through insulin receptors in fat cells. This process is accelerated by more vigorous exercise, but even low-level exercise is valuable, especially when starting from near zero. Parents are the "pep" team and should use their ingenuity to make exercise fun, with no hint of torture. Start slow and easy. . . but start!

Healthy Eating and Lifestyle

Too often, the evaluation of a diet is mainly based on its effectiveness in weight reduction. Low-fat diets are compared to low-carbohydrate diets. By zeroing in on fiber or omega-3 fats, considered singly, we have trouble seeing the forest for the trees. Diet superstars such as Barry Sears, Dean Ornish, and Robert C. Atkins have a single dietary principle attached to their names. The truth is they all have a lot to offer if we look at *all* they offer. For example, a look at Dr. Atkins' books, such as *Atkins for Life,* should dispel the myth that he wants you to load up on fat for the rest of your life. This misunderstanding is firmly planted in people's minds, but he only starts out with that regimen.[5] His no-carbohydrate recommendation is designed to act

DON'T GIVE IN TO QUICK FIXES

Even when being overweight is allowed to progress to "morbid obesity," one should avoid the temptation of the quick (but unhealthy) methods of weight-reducing medicines or surgery. Some of these medicines have been shown to produce an unacceptable association with "cardiovascular event risk" and are being taken off the market. Bariatric surgery involves any of several procedures that drastically reduce the size of the stomach. It should be considered the last option for reversing obesity of childhood. There are stricter requirements for consideration of surgery for adolescents than for adults, such as not proceeding unless there is failure to lose weight after a six-month effort and the presence of serious problems such as diabetes, sleep apnea, heart disease, or significant psychosocial impairment. It is good that there is some hesitancy to rush in with the surgical solution, because when opting for surgery all other attempts to lose weight are abandoned.

Surgery's main benefit of restricting intake comes at a price: drastically reducing stomach volume reduces the area responsible for hydrochloric acid output and the secretion of intrinsic factor. Mineral absorption, notably calcium, is dependent on gastric acid, and a lack of hydrochloric acid could also lead to vitamin-deficiency diseases, such as pellagra (vitamin B_3 deficiency) and beri-beri (vitamin B_1 deficiency). Intrinsic factor is necessary for the absorption of vitamin B_{12}. Deficiency diseases of B_{12} include a severe type of anemia and neurologic disease, including dementia. Once the surgery is performed, dietary restrictions are even tighter than those prior to surgery. By greatly reducing stomach size, the goal of restricting caloric intake is achieved, but some defeat the purpose of the surgery by indulging in frequent, high-calorie snacks and failing to exercise.

as a rescue operation, for a short period, for those overweight people who already have diabetes. Dr. Atkins goes into great detail about good "carbs" (whole grains) and bad "carbs" (refined), and he states that "carbohydrates play an important role in any balanced diet."

Trying to achieve weight loss by starvation is effective in the short term, but it is detrimental for the long haul. Many teenaged girls, in order to look better (which could translate to better acceptance by their peers) have tried this approach. Their idea is reinforced when homework keeps them up late and when classes begin all too early. Unfortunately for them, breakfast is just that—breaking a fast—and necessary. It should never be skipped! Under the influence of circadian rhythms (the body's natural 24-hour rhythm), stress hormones are kicking in early in the morning and demanding fulfillment of the body's need for fuel.

Time for homework deserves thought. A well thought-out plan for scheduling homework should include eating, sleeping, and even recreation. If these activities are not regulated, normal rhythms of the body are upset. In a growing adolescent, adequate restorative sleep is essential. Without it, there is restricted growth hormone production and sleep deprivation, associated with weight gain and poor concentration. There are, of course, individual variations for sleep need. Apply the "zombie vs. dynamo" test as your child approaches the breakfast table. "Zombies" need more sleep, so turn off the TV or disconnect that video game, pull out a storybook, and read them to sleep—any age-appropriate action to promote adequate sleep is a healthy idea.

Without breakfast, glucose from the liver and muscles is released and insulin is put into play to make it into usable, quick energy. These emergency stores are soon used up while insulin continues its action to store fat. It is as if the body says, "Since no food is available, I'd better go into conservation mode." Breakfast is the best meal for considering a solid protein intake that prevents the continuation of this problem as well as a "fuzzy brain" feeling later in the school morning. Eggs are an excellent source of protein as well of many other healthful nutrients. Check the color of the yolks—the more orange they are, the greater the antioxidant, vitamin, and other valuable nutrient content. Caged chickens will not have a source of these marvelous ingredients available to them, so look for a local, natural source for eggs from cage-free chickens.

Minimize your child's intake of refined carbohydrates, including white flour, sugar, and especially high-fructose corn syrup. Remember that sugars are soluble and are drunk as well as eaten and that soft drinks are loaded with sugars. A soft drink combined with a pastry is a double whammy. In small amounts, refined sugars and starches do not cause as much mischief as long as they are combined with fiber, a protein source, or fat. To break a habit of frequent huge servings of sugary soft drinks, it may be necessary to go cold turkey for a while and then reintroduce soda with a new look—as a rare luxury. Any food, such as potatoes, that is readily broken down into glucose should be eaten only in moderate amounts and with a look at its own fiber content (eat the skins) or if it is eaten with other stick-to-the-ribs foods. Apple juice does not pass the fiber test, whereas eating the whole apple does. It might take some doing to switch from white bread or pasta to partially whole grain, but it could prove surprising how tasty these previously avoided foods are.

An honest look at individual fats finds that some are not all that bad and some are necessary to sustain life. The anti-inflammatory value of omega-3 fatty acids (in cold-water fish) and the pro-inflammatory omega-6 fatty acids (many of the vegetable oils) must be considered. We need some of each group, so the solution is to reduce the ratio of omega-6s to omega-3s. You can be certain that wild salmon is rich in omega-3s, but not as certain about farmed fish. Some fish farms feed their fish with cheaper grains (omega-6 sources) as opposed to omega-3-rich algae from the sea. Fish oil capsules are an acceptable alternative for the real thing. Since butter and the predominant fatty acids of lard are saturated fats, they are already hydrogenated and resistant to oxidation. It is oxidation of polyunsaturated fats that produces harmful substances. Butter, consisting of short-chain fatty acids, has some other unique health benefits. These much-maligned fats should be thought of as condiments that, used in relatively small portions, can add zest to ordinary foods. Trans-fats, on the other hand, are foreign to our bodies and should not be eaten.

Vitamins and Other Supplements

Obesity, like no other childhood disorder, affects many aspects of health. Vitamin supplements will boost healthy metabolic pathways. All children need to take a daily vitamin-mineral preparation in order to supply nutrients that are lacking in an unattainable "perfect" diet. This can be in the form of a chewable tablet until the less expensive pill form can be swallowed.

Vitamin C—Take a minimum of one or two 500 mg chew-tabs daily. But you should also regard vitamin C as a medicine for specific needs, such as combating allergies and infections, prior to immunization administration, and counteracting other forms of stress. Vitamin C is a cofactor in numerous coenzymes, so intake must not be neglected. Because the vitamin is water soluble and is not stored in the body, C is best taken in divided doses throughout the day. Depending on age (size), if these forms of stress are more or less continuous, give 1,000 mg three times a day. At times of acute stress, determine the dose by the bowel tolerance rule. This is a variable individual determination, measured by noticing the dosage when loose stools occur; reduce the dose a bit when this condition is apparent. Depending on severity of the stress, the optimal dose might be quite high. What works for one child might not be appropriate for another, but we reassert that high doses of vitamin C are safe for all.

B Vitamins—The value of B vitamins is in their ubiquitous presence, as cofactors of coenzymes. We mentioned the huge role that niacin (B_3) plays in the "energy" (Krebs) cycle; extreme vitamin B deficiencies are reflected in many serious diseases, many of which (pellagra, beriberi) were known before pinning down the specific deficiency. Thiamine (B_1) is a co-factor in the enzyme pyruvate dehydrogenase, which gets derivatives of carbohydrates, amino acids, and fats into the cycle of energy production. Pyridoxine (B_6) plays a major part in many metabolic pathways and it has been shown to exhibit wide individual requirements. For example, up to twenty-five times the adult Recommended Dietary Allowance (RDA) may be needed to stop convulsions in a B_6-deficient infant. B_6 is getting popular attention for its role in neurotransmitter formation. We need not be concerned about the optimal dose of a specific B vitamin, however. A "B-50" preparation is readily available in the supermarket or drug store, and it contains 50 mg of the major B family and 50 micrograms (mcg) of those that are prescribed in smaller doses. The only noticeable side effect is that of voiding very yellow urine, colored by riboflavin (B_2). Better too much of these totally harmless vitamins than too little.

Vitamin E—It is practically impossible to get an adequate amount of vitamin E from the diet alone, even when in normal good health. Avocado is considered a good food source, yet it probably has just enough to prevent hydroperoxidation (a very unhealthy event) of the rich polyunsaturated fatty acid content of the fruit. With the bloodstream often loaded with fats in the obese, I recommend taking up to 800 IU of natural (d-alpha tocopherol) once daily. All children (without obesity) ages twelve through adolescence should be given 400 IU per day. Taking a fat-soluble vitamin only once a day is fine as long as it is with a meal. The natural E is 50 percent more efficient than the synthetic (d,l-alpha tocopherol).

Vitamin D—D is normally not specifically recommended for obesity, but we think that it is beneficial. Through its calcium regulation, vitamin D affects insulin target tissues and insulin resistance. During the recent H1N1 (swine) influenza epidemic, young people were hit extra hard, more than the older age group that usually suffers the most. Most of the deaths of children were of obese children, putting suspicion on defective immune systems that allowed the virus to create direct lung damage. On the other hand, it was found that infection with influenza virus and secondary problems were greatly reduced in non-vaccinated children who took high amounts of vitamin D (1,200 mg of D_3). Many illustrations of vitamin D's effect on the immune system can be found. The RDA is creeping up and may get to a good level eventually, but I see no reason to wait. Any child capable of swallowing a tiny pill should take 1,000 mg daily.

Selenium—The mineral selenium is not necessarily recommended for prevention or treatment of obesity, but it has an essential function in making glutathione, the powerful antioxidant. It seems to duplicate some vitamin E action, thus sparing vitamin E for other functions. Selenium has a stimulating effect on the immune system as shown by its deficiency causing some mediocre viruses to become truly bad actors (Coxsackie virus). Take 200 mcg a day. Whole grains are a good source, but many soils are deficient, making the food source uncertain.

Essential Fatty Acids—Pay special attention to the omega-6 to omega-3 ratio of foods; reduce your intake of the former and increase the latter. It might seem counter-productive recommending eating fatty fish, but due to its good fat content, a small serving goes a long way toward satisfying your appetite. If your child hasn't yet acquired a taste for fish, fish oil capsules are a good alternative. A typical preparation contains 1,000–1,200 mg of fish oil per capsule, and two capsules provide 750 mg of EPA (eicosapentaenoic acid) and DHA (docosahexaenoic acid), the two desirable long-chain fatty acids. These fatty acids dampen inflammation and lower triglycerides, and they appear to be effective in a relatively small dose. A capsule with breakfast and again with the noon meal would be good (if school makes the noon dose difficult, switch it to the evening meal). The capsules are big, so some creativity may be needed to get the contents ingested. Try opening each end of the capsule with a needle puncture and squeeze the contents into a small serving of orange juice. The monounsaturated oils (olive, peanut, and canola) can be considered better than neutral. Generally, olive oil is superior, as it undergoes less undesirable processing, and extra-virgin oil is cold pressed (no solvents) and contains some natural "super antioxidants." But it does have a pungent flavor that might make the others more preferable for some applications. Also, high temperatures harm olive oil, so do not fry with it. Use peanut oil instead, as it handles the heat well.

SUMMARY

Such a striking contrast in looking at pictures of high school students of a generation ago and students of the present age! There is a large discrepancy in the current population between the "fit" and the over-weight, making us ask which is normal? "Average" does not equate with "normal." Why have we allowed obesity to become such a problem? We have, through apathy and tolerance, simply denied that we know the root cause: faulty nutrition, with failure to avoid an excess intake of calories or participate in exercise to burn them. Obesity and type 2 diabetes go hand in hand as disorders prevented and treated by nutritional means. Stay away from medical and surgical remedies, and get on the right track. The rewards of weight control are much more far reaching.

CHAPTER 9

ALLERGIES AND ASTHMA

"One-quarter of what you eat keeps you alive.
The other three-quarters keeps your doctor alive."
—ATTRIBUTED TO HIEROGLYPHS FOUND IN
AN ANCIENT EGYPTIAN TOMB

Allergies and asthma are two subjects that strike close to home for me (RC). The old adage "It takes one to know one" certainly applies in my personal experiences with allergy-related problems. I had such severe nasal allergies as a junior high school student that there were times that I sounded like I had a clothespin clamping shut my nose. Thank goodness for a speech teacher who threatened to clobber anyone who made fun of me. I had heard that proper alignment of teeth in a growing person could only come about if the mouth remained closed during sleep. So, I had a choice: a nice smile or death by suffocation. I trained myself to keep my teeth properly aligned while I breathed with pursed lips even when sleeping.

At the same time, I intuitively discovered that a "healthful" (large size) glass of orange juice at breakfast not only made me woozy but stuffed up my nose. The stuffiness was also noted after drinking cow's milk. Fortuitously, I discovered that I could eat aged cheddar cheese with impunity, so this became my substitute for milk. An extra dividend that accrued was the development of strong, cavity-free teeth.

The good news is that allergies, if properly managed, may disappear with the passage of time. The bad news is that the tendency for allergy problems is often genetic. But, as with other inherited tendencies, one's fate is not sealed by simply making a diagnosis. Having my own children go through some allergy problems aided my ability to help other children.

In this chapter, we will examine the most prevalent types of allergies in children: gastrointestinal (food) allergies, hay fever, eczema, and asthma.

ALLERGENS AND ALLERGY DIAGNOSIS

Certain children, after being exposed to protein substances called allergens—by eating, by breathing, or by receiving an injection or contacting the allergen—become allergic to the allergen and express their allergy in various symptoms. The major classes of allergens are:

Food Allergens

In infants, commonly the proteins of cows' milk, wheat, orange juice, and egg whites cause allergies. In older children, these plus chocolate, onions, fish, pork, and nuts are the most common allergens, but most any food can be an allergen. A very common allergen is sucrose (table sugar). Food allergens may produce symptoms within 15 minutes after eating them (hay fever, hives, angioneurotic edema) up to twelve or more hours later (eczema flare-ups, asthma).

I discussed the prevalence of food allergy with a horticulturist at the beginning of the "organic" movement. He convinced me that applying too much chemical nitrogen to the soil of food crops causes the formation of abnormal proteins. I was very allergic to strawberries at that time, but his strawberries were perfectly innocuous. Abnormal proteins can be formed in plants in which too much inorganic nitrogen (chemical fertilizer) has been applied to the soil.

Inhalants

The most common inhalant allergens are the following:

- House dust, consisting of kapok, wool, feathers, and horsehair (from rug pads). Dust mites are also a contributing factor.

- Pollens of grasses, trees, and other plants.

- Animal danders from cats, dogs, and other pets. Dander may contribute to house dust as well.

- Molds.

With asthma, it may not come down to a single allergen or type of allergen. Rather, we need to look at several possible causes of bronchospasm and heavy secretions: viral or bacterial infection, exercise-induced exacerbation, or airborne pollutants and irritants (chemicals, particulate matter).

One of the pioneers in pediatric allergy problems, Dr. William Deamer, formed the concept of "allergy load." And pediatric allergist Dr. William Crook spoke of "hidden allergies." It is essential to pin down the cause of severe allergy reactions, and severe reactions often are caused by only one antigen, making detection a bit easier. Also, the antigenic culprit in a severe allergic reaction often can be identified with specific tests (such as measuring IgE antibodies in blood). Milder forms of allergy (hidden allergies) do not have that specificity and could involve several sensitivities causing the same manifestation—representing an "allergy load." For example, a person is allergic to a grass pollen, orange juice, and cat dander. On a bad day, when other factors are attacking the immune system, exposure to only one of these may set off symptoms (such as hay fever). On other days, it may take two or even all three exposures to do the same. We might not be able to identify every culprit, but eliminating any of the allergens will reduce the allergy load and improve symptoms.

It has taken about three decades to find agreement among allergists that allergens that are identified by "scratch" tests, "prick" tests, or measurement of IgE antibodies in the blood are not the only kinds of food allergens. Dr. Crook's "hidden food allergens" are based on a different immune response: through the formation of IgG antibodies. Laboratory testing is expensive and impractical. Ultimately, the only useful testing is through food challenges, because we are more interested in what allergens do to the body than in how they affect test results.

Observing the relationship of contact with the allergen and the production of symptoms is the only practical method of detecting food allergens. It is easier to relate immediate symptoms to the allergen than delayed symptoms. For example, in a child with eczema, if orange juice caused eczema and a runny nose, it will be easier to note its effect on the nose than on the skin. If the child goes to the dinner table free of allergy signs and symptoms and leaves the table showing many of the signs, there's a clear link. While it is fresh in your mind, write a list of everything your child has had to eat and drink. Several such lists can be cross-checked and some suspicious allergens found. Be sure to list individual ingredients: instead of "spaghetti," write "tomato, onion, beef, egg, wheat," and so on.

Better than any expensive laboratory test or diagnostic skin testing is the "elimination-and-challenge" method. This time-honored, inexpensive approach pins down what an allergen does in the *body*, not just in the laboratory or in the doctor's office. Suspected allergens derived from the food diary are eliminated. If you are short on suspects, eliminate items from the common "hidden food allergies" group, such as cow's milk, sugar, wheat, and orange juice. If your suspicions are correct, symptoms should be relieved within a few days. Then begin adding back one food at a time to identify the culprit (or culprits). If a particular food item is, indeed, an allergen, symptoms will flare up; otherwise, symptoms will not be present. Wait two to three days before testing other suspected allergens. If results are ambiguous, continue the food diary to search for further suspects.

GASTROINTESTINAL ALLERGIES

Forceful vomiting in a newborn raises a red flag to consider a diagnosis of pyloric stenosis. The pylorus is the intestinal end of the stomach, fitted with a muscular ring around it that acts as a valve (also referred to as the pylorus) to enable the stomach to retain its contents long enough to complete its part of digestion. "Stenosis" refers to narrowing. Diagnosis is completed by skillfully feeling the enlarged olive-shaped pylorus. The solution is surgical slitting of the muscular ring—easy for the skilled surgeon but tough on parents. I feel that food allergy, from proteins in the amniotic fluid, could well be the reason for the muscle hypertrophy. This is hard to confirm, because rarely is allergy management allowed a trial period before rushing into surgery. And, in at least one case I had, the surgery provided life-saving relief, but some gastrointestinal allergy symptoms persisted.

The appearance of mucus (without the bad odor of infectious diarrhea) or blood flecking in the stool indicates severe disease. Food allergy usually develops after prolonged exposure (a few weeks) to a food allergen. The newborn can be affected by allergens in mother's milk due to the mother's own sensitivity, most commonly a sensitivity to cow's milk. Perhaps the mother didn't show any of her own manifestations of being allergic to cow's milk, yet her infants were allergic to her breast milk and were relieved when she discontinued cow's milk in her diet.

If an anal rash is localized and itchy (the older child can show you), it is similar to contact dermatitis. Some allergen in the stool is causing this skin reaction. If the rash is widespread in the diaper area and solid "deep red," it more likely is due to thrush, a yeast infestation of the gut, seen in an older infant.

We hear a lot about irritable bowel syndrome (and its medical relief) in adults. In infants, it can be manifest as either constipation or diarrhea. In adults, emotional stress has to be considered as a cause, but adults with this syndrome should also look at the allergy hypothesis before turning to medications, which could mask the symptoms and make allergy detection impossible. And the flip side: Could a screaming, uncomfortable baby get its bowels in an uproar? I think so.

Severe gastrointestinal allergy must be dealt with promptly. The infant must be able to retain and gain sustenance from ingested water and nourishment. If forceful vomiting has continued for even a short time, the infant should receive medical attention. The smaller the infant, the less its tolerance for dehydration and starvation. Water by mouth, if retained, could lead to a trial of a hydrolyzed protein formula, in which the milk proteins are broken down into their respective amino acids, disabling the protein's allergenic potential. Feedings or water should be offered in small amounts initially, while gradually increasing the volume and time interval between feedings.

At the same time, the child's doctor may decide to administer methyl scopolamine nitrate, a drug that relaxes the muscle of the pylorus. I have witnessed a pyloric "tumor" fade away under this treatment, but the drug might no longer be available. At any rate, the attending doctor would need to be willing to try this. If the baby is dehydrated, immediate surgery and intravenous fluids would be the more likely course of action.

After surgical relief, the infant's parents can start oral feedings with hypoallergenic formula in the immediate postoperative period. With adequate weight gain and other evidences of thriving, a switch to a less expensive soy formula can be made. (In time, soy can prove to be sensitizing just like cow's milk, but this might take several months.) If the infant's condition is good, a challenge with a small amount of a regular cow's milk formula could be tried. If vomiting recurs, go back to feeding with the hypoallergenic formula and stay away from cow's milk for several months.

Up to this point, I have not mentioned anything about breastfeeding because forceful vomiting in the breastfed infant is rare. However, intact milk proteins can escape digestion in some nursing mothers, sneak from her gut into the bloodstream, and pass through in her breast milk. This is often referred to as the "leaky gut syndrome." It will not pose a threat to the newborn, but after a period of sensitization, it could cause problems later on. Severe gastrointestinal symp-

Symptoms of Gastrointestinal Allergies in Infants

- Vomiting (forcefully rather than just "spitting up")
- Cramping and colic, with mucus in the stool, loose stools, and sometimes blood flecks in the mucus in the stools
- Rash around anus (sometimes extending to the buttocks) with itching
- Hard, pellet-like stools rather than loose stools (in older infants and children)

toms that come on immediately after birth must represent prenatal sensitization from the mother's leaky gut syndrome. The fetus is sensitized through the conjoined blood circulation and I would think from swallowed amniotic fluid.

Mucus in the stool, especially if accompanied with blood flecks or stringy strands of blood, represents severe sensitization. Without vomiting, the infant might tolerate fairly normal feedings of a hydrolysate formula. If there is evidence of bleeding, the gut is badly damaged and recovery requires very careful management. Without such management, there is the danger of developing a new, severe sensitivity. Let months go by before challenging with any of the usual food allergen culprits.

HAY FEVER (NASAL ALLERGIES)

Sinuses are literally holes in the head. As far as I can see, their main functions are to add resonance to the speaking voice and increase the strength of the facial bones. The openings (ostia) of the sinuses drain into the nasal cavity. Their lining, like the mucous membranes of the nose, can secrete mucus or worse material if infection is present. Allergy, infection, or airborne irritants can cause inflammatory swelling of the openings, causing retention of those secretions. The effect is a change in the quality of the voice (a "sinusy" voice).

In front of a mirror, tilt your head back. Push up the tip of your nose and you will see a mound of tissue on each side, coming from the side and projecting toward the nasal septum in the middle. Those are the lowest of three turbinates, bony projections covered with mucus. If a person is allergic to a grass pollen, when the pollen adheres to the mucous membranes, it will create an outpouring of mucus, accompanied by itching. Strangely enough, these tissues can also respond to allergens in the bloodstream, such as food allergens. A child with allergic rhinitis (hay fever) often exhibits the "allergic salute," a rapid motion in which the back of the hand pushes up the tip of the nose. This is accompanied by an annoying (in the ears of the beholder), audible sniff as the excess mucus is pulled into the throat while attempting to scratch the itch in the nose and throat.

When lying down, it is even harder for secretions to get out the narrowed "front door," creating postnasal drip. Tissues in the back of the throat are irritated from the constant bombardment of postnasal drip and become a sort of trigger center for a "tickly," dry cough. If secretions accumulate, then a cough might sound "rattly"

SYMPTOMS OF NASAL ALLERGIES

- A stopped-up nose with "nasal" voice, snoring, and mouth breathing
- "Itchy" nose—rubbed often or red (or red, itchy eyes) and frequent sneezing
- "Runny" nose—with clear, thin mucus nasal discharge or white nasal discharge
- Constant sniffling, or a perpetual annoying (to parents) dry cough—worse when lying down (postnasal drip)
- Rattling cough that sounds like it is in the chest because of vibration in throat transmitted throughout the chest
- "Colds" that last weeks rather than days
- History of frequent "colds" with or without fever; many ear infections in infancy, or need for adenoidectomy by three years of age
- A pale appearance about the face, dark circles under eyes (due to partially blocked lymphatic drainage), or puffy areas under the eyes (at lower outer corners of eyes)
- "Sinus trouble" in adults
- Chronic sore, dry throat, or hoarseness noted after arising in the morning
- Granular eyelids (sandy feeling in the eyes)
- Itching in throat and ears after eating a food allergen (if itching is also in bloodshot eyes, some allergen in the air, such as grass pollen, is the troublemaker)

and can be confused with a productive cough that emanates from the bronchi. It is analogous to striking the top of a chime and feeling the blow transmitted down the tube. A rattling cough with its origin in the throat can actually be felt in the chest.

Watery eyes are due to the tear ducts being blocked at the nasal end. The duct is enclosed in that little bump in the nasal corner of the eye. Its purpose is to act as a drain for tears. An older child with allergy to airborne pollens may show the signs of allergic conjunctivitis: itchy, slightly bloodshot eyes. On inspection of a turned down lower eyelid, there is the appearance of red bumps that resemble a cobblestone road.

Food allergens in infants and preschoolers may cause a "tension-fatigue" syndrome that is often associated with nasal allergy. The child at times doesn't act like himself—he is extremely restless and whiney, easily frustrated, and will cry and scream over nothing— while you, the parent, feel that you cannot get "through" to him for love or money.

In most infants, nasal allergy is usually manifested by noisy breathing. A consistently itchy, runny nose in a toddler is the signal to get going on the detective work on all fronts: food allergens, chemicals, and inhalants such as house dust, molds, and pollens. The nasal allergy signs related to food or drink sensitivity occur quickly after ingestion. If the child does not have allergy symptoms when first sitting down to a meal, and very shortly after nasal allergy symptoms arise, write down everything the child ate or drank at that time (the "observation" protocol). Observation can also pin down many inhalant allergens. For example, if being around the cat or in a room that was just vacuumed brings on nasal allergy symptoms, think of cat dander and dust mite sensitivity. In the case of sensitivity to dander, the cat must, at the very least, be kept out of the room where the child spends the most time.

Dust mite sensitivity presents an interesting picture. Looking at a mite under the microscope reveals something resembling a fearsome crab. The crab itself doesn't cause harm but its excretions do. Dust mites love to inhabit the nap of carpet or a throw rug. This sensitivity would be suspected if a toddler or older child shows nasal allergy signs when playing on this surface. If a considerable reaction occurs a number of times, the dust mite must be turned out of its home by removing the floor covering and getting down to a hard surface, and by encasing bedding that can't be washed regularly in dust-proof material. Anything that is soft and can be brought near the nose also has to go. To avoid psychological trauma, be prepared to substitute a desirable mite-proof (and allergen-free) bedtime friend for the current favorite. The mattress cover for the older child's bed will be better accepted if a mattress pad that can be easily washed in hot water is used under the bottom sheet. If the floor covering must stay, use a vacuum cleaner that has a dust and pollen filter, and keep your child out of the room for several hours after vacuuming.

Mold sensitivity that begins in the older child is brought to attention more often in those with asthma. Many times, a musty odor is a give-away. Outdoors, the onset of mold season often begins in the fall before a heavy frost occurs, so avoiding stirring up decaying vegetation might be all that is necessary. In damp areas inside, such as in a basement, look for a white coating on windowsills. This can be treated with a fifty-fifty solution of chlorine bleach and water, if your child is not overly sensitive to chlorine. When avoidance is not sufficient and the symptoms are considerably more than simply annoying, desensitization through an allergist might be in order. A terrible situation has arisen in recent years. Severe mold growth is occurring in some newly built homes that have used foreign-made gypsum in sheetrock, the stuff of interior walls. There were questions of whether the material was faulty or just had been subjected to too much mold-supporting moisture. At any rate, hidden destruction of the structure took place, and the inhabitants have suffered from severe respiratory disease.

In older children, pollen sensitivity may be suspected as the cause of allergic symptoms, especially when other family members suffer from this. Since the problem is seasonal, one can usually get by with simple solutions until the season is over. The differentiating symptom of inhalant sensitivity is the itchy eyes that result from the inhalant getting into the eyes as well as the nose. A tangible example is sensitivity to one of the tall grasses. Running through a field of grass brings on sneezing, copious amounts of clear nasal mucus, and itchy eyes. If contact with this grass is unavoidable, protect your child against it by having him or her wear dark glasses, a cap, and a paper facemask. Afterwards, use eyedrops to flush pollen from the eyes, and shampoo to rid pollen residue from the hair. A nasal flush, for an older child, can get any pollen out of the nose that sneaked past the barrier. (For the flush, prepare a solution of one-quarter teaspoon of table salt in 8 ounces of warm water. Pour some into the cupped hand and vigorously sniff it through the nose into the throat. Pinch off one nostril at a time and blow the contents out. Repeat this two or three times.)

Any sudden allergy attack indicates that there is a sudden release of histamine causing the symptoms. Histamine is neutralized by vitamin C. There is no harm from a high dose of vitamin C, so start with 2,000 mg for a child weighing over 45 pounds. If this is effective, the amount can be reduced the next time, as you find the lowest effective dose. If symptoms persist until bedtime, despite attempts at washing away lingering pollen, a simple, reliable antihistamine like Chlortrimeton can be used. I have not seen more drowsiness from Chlortrimeton than from newer antihistamines, and a little drowsiness at bedtime isn't a bad idea. This is not intended to be other than a short-term, nighttime solution. Vitamin C can be used liberally in the daytime and may be completely effective, eliminating the need for an antihistamine.

SKIN MANIFESTATIONS OF ALLERGY

Eczema is also called infantile eczema, atopic dermatitis, and nummular dermatitis (from a Latin word meaning "coin"). It is said to occur in infants less than six months of age (though I have never seen this), and it can be a real problem in the older infant and toddler age group. Eczema typically appears as a red rash over the cheeks, in back of the knees, and in the folds of the elbows, and it can itch intensely. Damage to the skin from scratching changes the appearance; little bumps or blisters that weep when broken add to the picture.

Some feel the itching of eczema results from fluid buildup in the deeper layer of skin. I learned from a pediatric dermatologist that "eczema is an itch that rashes." This made sense when he also told us about the "white scratch test": if you scratch the smooth skin of the underside of your forearm with your fingernail and wait a few seconds, a red flare should appear where you scratched. If you are prone to eczema, a white streak appears. There must be some link between the nerves that relay the "itch" message to the brain and the skin they supply.

The principle cause of eczema is one or more food sensitivities. Proceed with detective work, via the "elimination and challenge" method, to identify the culprit(s). Other environmental factors need to be considered, as well. At bath time, do not use hot water, and use a hypoallergenic soap only sparingly. Some strongly recommend using only what are called "emollients," which soften and soothe the skin, in place of soap (ask your pharmacist). Instead of rough toweling off, pat dry. Avoid clothing next to the skin made from rougher or scratchier materials like wool; cotton "breathes" better and is smoother. When a person with eczema becomes overheated, sweating can make the itching more intense.

Because the inflamed skin in eczema is like an open wound, you will need to be on the alert for infection. An early *Streptococcus* infection will look something like raw beefsteak; *Staphylococcus* produces little pus-filled blisters. Both will intensify the itching. These infections need immediate attention. While investigating possible food allergens and taking other preventive measures, itching can produce discomfort that causes sleeplessness. So while you are investigating possible food allergens and taking other preventive measures in order to find a more permanent solution, liquid Benadryl given at bedtime will help relieve itching when used sparingly in the short term. If there are no signs of infection and little weeping, cool (not warm, not cold) compresses gently laid on the area often provide relief from itching.

Hives and angioneurotic edema are much more serious. The latter condition needs immediate medical attention should it occur. Hoarseness is the sign of imminent life-threatening laryngospasm (the larynx closes, completely blocking the airway).

SYMPTOMS OF ECZEMA

- In infants, a rash over the cheeks, front of elbows, and back of knees; it is red and itches, but varies from being dry (in the more chronic stage) to weeping and oozing (in the more acute stage)

- In older children, often just dry, scaly, itchy coin-sized patches

Skin Manifestations

- Hives—red, raised welts with white centers; they itch

- Angioneurotic edema is a hive-like rash but much worse, with life-threatening symptoms—puffy lips and eyes, with sudden onset of becoming pale (sometimes with a hoarse cough); often "giddy" or in a cold sweat

Eczema represents severe allergy sensitivity and demands the use of similar vitamin and mineral supplements as used for asthma. In addition to the basic multivitamin-mineral preparation (in age-related appropriate form), plus the vitamin extras recommended for all children, more is needed for these two stress-producing disorders. For one too young to manage a chewtab form of supplement, powdered or crystalline vitamin C (1,000 mg; a quarter teaspoonful) can be added to juice (non-allergenic) or to a little honey in water; dispense 500 mg or more, three times a day. An older child can take 1,000 mg three times a day in the form of 500-mg chewtabs or crystalline C. This amount should be tolerated well. If stools become loose, back off the dose a bit. These are preventive doses that can be increased during illness; bowel tolerance of vitamin C is the upper limit.

In addition to vitamin C, some yogurt each day is helpful, along with vitamins A, D, and E and no junk food. It sounds like a truism, but the way to end skin problems is to have healthy skin. While a long way from an instant eczema cure (of which there are none), the nutritional route is well worth trying.

PREVENTION AND SYMPTOM RELIEF FOR ALLERGIES

Essential Fatty Acids

Why consider these essential fatty acids? Increasing the intake of omega-3 fatty acids and reducing the intake of omega-6 fatty acids can reduce the inflammatory response. Essential fatty acids are the progenitors of prostaglandins, which reside in cell membranes, as if on alert, ready to perform their actions when needed. Prostaglandins are lipid compounds derived from fatty acids that mediate a number of physiological effects, including constriction or dilation of vascular smooth muscle cells, bronchoconstriction or dilation, aggregation or disaggregation of platelets (clotting), and regulation of inflammation. Some prostaglandins have a normalizing effect (the "good" prostaglandins), while others lead to abnormal function (the "bad" prostaglandins). Ultimately, all prostaglandins are derived from arachidonic acid, which also is the forerunner of inflammation builders called leukotrienes.

Prostaglandin E_2 (PGE_2) has an inhibitory effect on some products favorable for our immune systems, while allowing the production of things that are detrimental. It is one of the main producers of inflammation. In the newborn, PGE_2 leads to an allergy-producing immune reaction and production of IgE antibodies (the humoral immune response), a process initiated in the fetus. But to protect the newborn from viral and bacterial infection, the immune response has to shift to the other type, the innate response, involving T cells. So, early exposure to infectious agents will hasten this shift and will reduce the prospect of allergy problems later.

For about the first six months of life, the infant does not make the enzyme that leads down the good prostaglandin production path.[1] The good news is that breast milk can provide an adequate amount of it. This is certainly a reason for encouraging breastfeeding as well as an explanation of why breastfeeding guards against infectious diseases of infancy. Besides these dietary inadequacies that have altered our immune system health, the diminished intake of antioxidants the over past thirty years provides more oxidative stress and a shift to more inflammation.

Aspirin and similar drugs are used for relieving inflammation that is a part of many diseases. Aspirin inhibits the enzyme that stimulates production of all prostaglandins. It is effective because bad prostaglandins have a much stronger action than the weaker, good prostaglandins. But by stopping production of all prostaglandins, the good as well as the bad, long-term aspirin use creates other unanticipated problems. Ironically, aspirin sensitivity is fairly common in those with asthma and can trigger the formation of nasal polyps in those with nasal allergy, which almost completely block the nasal airway.

Omega-6 fatty acids, depending on the enzymes involved, form both bad prostaglandins (such as thromboxane, which causes clumping of platelets and constriction of arteries) and good ones. An omega-3 fatty acid, the fish oil eicosapentaenoic acid (EPA), inhibits a step that leads to the production of bad rather than good prostaglandins, while insulin stimulates this production. From this, we can see that a diet high in refined carbohydrates that raises insulin levels interferes with our attempt to quell inflammation. Some good but relatively weak prostaglandins are also built from EPA. Overall, we want to inhibit the building of bad prostaglandins from arachidonic acid. Reducing omega-6s while increasing omega-3s is a direct way of favorably influencing prostaglandin production and inflammation.

Water

Your body is mostly water. Water can be good for what ails you. Drink a lot of water and you will feel better immediately: headaches vanish, stuffiness clears up, your gastrointestinal "plumbing" will work like a dream (less constipation, risk of kidney stones drops to near zero), and it will even help you lose a bit of weight (especially in combination with vegetable juicing). Do not take this as an excuse or an endorsement to spend money on water products, with the possible exception of an inexpensive device to clean up your drinking water if you live in an area where tap water is a bit dicey.

I (AWS) am talking about drinking water by the glassful. Don't limit your fluids unless there is a clear medical requirement for doing so. Open the hatch and gulp it down! It is remarkably difficult to overhydrate yourself, but it is amazingly easy to get dehydrated. Though everyone knows that hot weather activity causes water loss, you need as much or more to replace water lost in cold weather activity. It is not just exercising that causes water loss: talking uses water (classroom teachers need an extra liter or two a day) and airline travel dehydrates you. Certainly the value is great, the safety high, and the price is right.

President Ronald Reagan's personal physician, Ralph Bookman, M.D., simply told the president to drink a good bit more water to relieve allergies. There's a good idea in general, and it's drug-free. In an interview, Dr. Bookman said, "Unquestionably, the single most important element in the treatment of asthma and other bronchial allergy symptoms is hydration. Unless adequate fluids are available to the mucous glands in the bronchial tree, their secretions will be tenaciously hard to raise. In asthma, liquids are medications. Liquids make mucus liquid. They change it from a troublesome solid that makes breathing difficult to an easy to cough up liquid. I demand that my patients drink ten full glasses of liquid every day, and I question them constantly to make sure they understand how important it is."[2]

Naturally, we certainly do *not* recommend ten glasses of water a day for all children, regardless of size! I (RC) always gauge adequate hydration by the color of the urine (after the morning riboflavin is flushed away). Children often need reminders to take on water, but not a set amount. The bronchial secretions in asthma are of a very "ropy" consistency, not easily broken up with water intake alone. I have found grapefruit juice to be the best children's expectorant.

Vitamin C

A young woman, age twenty, was brought to see me (AWS) once by her family. She was allergic to horses and hay. Since she loved to ride, and her parents kept several horses in their barn, this was a big problem. The young lady was not readily going to change her eating habits, but was willing to take a lot of vitamin C. It was effective, as she tells it: "Whenever I was taking 20,000 milligrams of vitamin C a day, I had no allergies at all. The only time I got them back was when I drank beer. So I either avoided beer or, if I drank, I took an extra 10,000 mg of C. I never had problems with horses or hay again."

I had another client once who was allergic to everything, literally. She said that she'd tested positive as allergic to seventy-two different substances. I'd never heard of that severe a condition before and, apparently, neither had her allergist. He said that she could take a "megadose" of perhaps 1,000 milligrams a day. It was not doing anything, so I suggested she take vitamin C to bowel tolerance, and hold the C level just below the amount that caused loose stools. This turned out to be nearly 40,000 mg a day. She took all the C she could hold, and that was the end of her allergies.

Take enough C to be symptom free, whatever the amount might be. Stay a few thousand milligrams under the amount that would cause loose bowels.

Some of what we now label "allergies" may often just as easily be called "undernutrition"—insufficient vitamin C results in exaggerated sensitivity to even average levels of irritants, toxins, chemicals, pollution, and microorganisms. Deficiencies of vitamins A, B-complex, and E frequently manifest as skin problems or hypersensitivity to foods, stress, germs, or shock. Millions of vitamin-deficient but overstuffed persons are waiting to be allergic to something. Food that fills and fattens but doesn't fortify the body is like trying to build a wall with bricks and no mortar: it will hold up only until you lean upon it.

Symptoms tell us that our body is not quite right. In that case, we should consider how we take care of it. Check your diet first, not only for the presence of allergens but rather for an absence of nutrients. (You can start with a saturation test with vitamin C, as mentioned above.) Are you avoiding chemical preservatives and other unnecessary food additives? Are you avoiding drugs, non-prescription and otherwise? Are you getting enough rest? Eating a whole-foods diet? These questions may go a long way toward ending battery after battery of allergy tests.

ASTHMA

Wheezing is a squeaking, musical sound produced when breathing out, and it is associated with difficult breathing. Breathing out is more laborious than breathing in, and often there is a "dry," unrelenting cough with wheezing. The noise, irregular in-and-out breathing, and dry (non-productive) cough are all due to bronchospasm. There is smooth muscle around the branches of the bronchi that is responsive to both the direct effect of inflammation from allergens or infectious agents and the nerve supply. Under the control of nerves from the sympathetic (autonomic) nervous system, the ring-like muscles can either contract to constrict the bronchus or relax to relieve the constriction. When constricted, air movement is difficult. On inspiration, the diaphragm creates a vacuum in the chest cavity that, if strong enough, allows air to flow in even when there is partial obstruction. Expiration is a more passive event. The diaphragm "pulls" but has little "push." With severe restriction, the muscles of the rib cage are brought into play to try to squeeze air out of the lungs—a very inefficient and exhausting help. This creates the jerky respiratory pattern of inspiration being faster than expiration. Bronchial constriction makes it difficult for bronchial secretions to be coughed up, leading to the ineffectual dry cough. As liquids are absorbed from the secretions, they become sticky with almost the consistency of glue.

No doctor or parent is anything other than uncomfortable when observing an infant or child having trouble with breathing. Nasal allergy may seem like just an annoying problem, but wheezing needs immediate attention. I am using the term *asthma* here for simplification. One is not said to have asthma unless there is some sense of

SYMPTOMS OF ASTHMA

- Wheezing with a cold (usually also with a fever)
- The majority of colds turn into "chest colds"
- Wheezing while not sick ("out of the blue")

chronicity to periods of bronchoconstriction and respiratory distress. Asthma may be due to a number of factors: allergies, exercise, irritants in the air, infectious causes of inflammation, or there may be an emotional, stressful component.

Wheezing in an infant or toddler poses a problem in diagnosis—namely, separating allergy from a viral infection. Every year, we have a round of respiratory syncytial virus (RSV), which presents as a flu-like illness with sinusitis in older children and adults (sometimes accompanied by a bloody nasal discharge and "raw," burning nose and sinus membranes) that is dismissed as "just another bad bug." Once had, partial immunity is afforded for the next year. Unfortunately, a newborn caught in an epidemic, with first-time exposure, can get seriously ill from bronchiolitis, inflammation of the small branches of the bronchial tree in which there are no muscles around them that might respond to bronchodilating medicines. RSV infection seems to make these infants prone in subsequent seasons to other virus-induced wheezing.

There are many viral infections that play a part in bronchoconstriction in susceptible individuals. This type of asthma can usually be managed well with a medicine to relieve (dilate) the constricted bronchi. Much of what we write here is advice on how to safely avoid running to the doctor and to thoughtfully consider the use of medicines. An infant or child with the appearance of asthma who is having real trouble breathing needs immediate medical attention, both for accurate diagnosis and treatment. Detective work to identify all possible "triggers" is the first, essential step.

Determine what is the most appropriate type of bronchodilator to have on hand. An older child may be able to handle an inhaler, whereas a younger one would need a liquid, oral preparation. Any of these medicines are most effective when used early on, as soon as the first signs of a "tight," dry cough or other difficulty with air exchange. Finding a dose that is effective without causing jitteriness (one of the main side effects) is reassuring to the patient, the parent, and the doctor. Soothing the uneasiness produced by finding it hard to get a breath as well as that from the anxiety-like effects of the medicine itself requires a calm, reassuring atmosphere. When the child is well is a good time to think about how one stays as calm as possible during an attack. Having success with nipping an attack in the bud is very reassuring. If an attack progresses to the point of real difficulty breathing, massaging the back muscles helps, as well as knowing that help is near if relief doesn't come soon.

Dr. Saul's Seven Ways to Avoid an Asthma Attack

1. Take vitamin C—Lack of vitamin C can cause asthma, high-dose vitamin C relieves it. Researchers have found that asthma is linked to both a decreased preference for foods containing vitamin C and lower concentrations of vitamin C in the blood.[3] Robert Cathcart, M.D., recommends a daily vitamin C (ascorbate) dosage of between 15,000 to 50,000 mg, divided into eight doses.[4] He writes: "Asthma is most often relieved by bowel tolerance doses of ascorbate. A child regularly having asthmatic attacks following exercise is usually relieved of these attacks by large doses of ascorbate. So far, all of my patients having asthmatic attacks associated with the onset of viral diseases have been ameliorated by this treatment." When consumed in regular, frequent, near-saturation-doses, vitamin C is a powerful antihistamine.[5]

   Once, my next-door neighbor's four-year-old boy got into his mom's vitamin C and ate about twenty tablets. He had no diarrhea or side effects at all, except that his asthma symptoms went away. The lesson here is Linus Pauling's: "Keep medicine out of the reach of everybody. Use vitamin C instead."

2. Stop smoking—Smoking around asthmatics should be considered assault, and smoking around children should be seen as child abuse. Smoking, or simply breathing second-hand tobacco smoke, destroys vitamin C. Do not allow asthmatics near smokers, and this goes double for children. It will not surprise anyone to learn that many scientific studies confirm the link between children's exposure to tobacco smoke and increased incidence of asthma.[6] Cigarette smoke causes asthma even before the child is born.[7] Total avoidance of second-hand smoke is a given for asthma management.

3. Reduce stress—Stress reduction greatly helps asthmatics, reducing airway resistance and decreasing the severity of symptoms.[8] Some research has reported profound improvement and a decreasing need for anti-asthmatic drugs.[9]

4. Straighten your spine, and keep your back in line—This may mean regular visits to a good chiropractor or it may mean yoga, regular exercise, and stretches every day. Although still controversial in medical circles, these simple measures may provide noticeable relief for asthma. The chiropractic profession has published a considerable number of preliminary studies and case reports suggesting that spinal manipulation benefits asthmatics. Great stress is put on the abdominal and lower back muscles when trying to squeeze out the air during an attack. Strengthening them is good.

5. Eat horseradish and cayenne pepper, and drink plenty of water—My grandfather was firefighter in the 1930s, long before respirators and other lung protection was available. He was overcome with smoke many times in the course of his dangerous career, saving lives at risk of his own lungs. The toll was asthma-like symptoms that became worse in later life. I remember him literally covering his food with cayenne pepper, and he ate horseradish, and even breathed the vapors, as first aid. It sounds odd, but he said it made his breathing easier, and I can tell you from being there that it apparently did.

6. Take homeopathic medicines—I think a look into homeopathic remedies for asthma is worth your time. There are a number of nonprescription, combination homeopathic remedies on the market. One might look into *Aconitum napthallus* (aconite), a microdilution of the monkshood herb. It is good first aid for an asthma attack. However, your taking lots of vitamin C may eliminate your need for even this natural remedy.

7. Try deep breathing—When a child is old enough to understand the basics of asthma, he or she should be reminded that the inhaler works best when used at the first sign of a "tight" chest or "dry" cough. When not wheezing, deep breathing should be done sever-

al times a day. This increases lung capacity and raises the threshold for bronchospasm. "Deep" breathing is abdominal breathing. Pull that diaphragm down as far as it will go while watching the abdomen swell. (Expanding the chest is not effective.) On the exhale phase, squeeze every last bit of air out of the lungs. Do six "in-and-outs" a session. At the beginning of an attack, deep breathing may abort it. Still, reach for the vitamin C.

Asthma Management

If asthma attacks are frequent, in spite of a diligent search for causative factors, and the first-line treatments are not adequate, management of the condition is much more difficult. The strongest anti-inflammatory drugs are cortisone derivatives. A shot of adrenaline is the rescue medicine that works quickly, while oral cortisone derivatives are part of more long-term treatment. Because of serious side effects from long-term use, parents and doctors need to work closely together to make this adjunct of management as short-term as possible.

House dust and molds in the air that bring on asthma attacks, and are not controlled by the measures described in the nasal allergy section, may require other methods of management. Room air filters that siphon out particulate matter (dust, pollens, molds) are available. If the house has forced-air heat, there are electric precipitators that can be installed into the heating unit. Particles are "charged" as they pass through, then precipitate on plates of the opposite charge; the plates can be removed and cleaned. If these measures fail to provide good control, desensitizing through the services of an allergist should be considered. Often, an allergist can work together with your personal doctor to avoid the confusion of not knowing whom to call when questions arise.

The subtle deterioration of the American diet over the past several decades is evidenced by the increase in the incidence of asthma, as well as its severity. The inflammation pathway is augmented by a marked decrease in the intake of antioxidants. Potent antioxidants found in vegetables and fruits are not as much a part of today's diet as they should be. Vitamin C is said to be the major respiratory antioxidant, and those with low levels have a five-fold increase in asthma incidence. Vitamin E is also strongly correlated with lung function,[10] and vitamin A has a strong influence on the health of cells that make up the respiratory tree lining. So, find the best acceptable diet available after eliminating sensitizing foods. Be sure to think of all the components of the eliminated food that should be included in the substitute food or as a supplement (for example, the calcium of cow's milk). Supplements of vitamins A, C, E, and D should be added to the vegetable- and fruit-rich basic diet at the earliest age possible. Levels of selenium-glutathione peroxidase, a strong antioxidant enzyme made in the body, can be enhanced by providing additional selenium. The mineral selenium also prevents stress-induced damage to immune cells.[11] If the child is not sensitive to fish, fish oil and its content of omega-3 fatty acids can provide relief from the inflammatory aspects of asthma. The huge capsules can be pricked at both ends and the contents squeezed into a non-allergic juice—one or two a day, depending on the size of the child.

SUMMARY

We have dealt with allergy problems by putting them into separate "signs and symptoms" categories, according to the area affected. Histamine release is responsible for swelling of membranes, excessive amounts of mucus, and itching—all very annoying. Of greater concern are the more serious conditions that can arise from immune system–mediated reactions: asthma, angioneurotic edema, and severe gastrointestinal symptoms.

In addition to identifying and eliminating all proven allergens, we should boost immune system function. More attention is being given to the inflammatory aspects of asthma and how, in infancy, the immune system can be influenced to follow the allergy route or the better pathway that defends against infection. More allergists are broadening their views and considering the part that food allergens and early, moderate exposure to an environment that is other than sterile might play. Old standards of thinking are falling, and better methods of diagnosis and treatment are slowly evolving.

Safe methods, such as large doses of vitamin C, along with the other vitamin supplement boosters mentioned in this chapter, certainly should be "first line" treatments. As you find your child's optimal and therapeutic amount of vitamin C, you will be able to phase out medical treatment. But don't do this abruptly, especially if on a medical regimen for severe asthma.

CHAPTER 10

ATTENTION-DEFICIT HYPERACTIVITY DISORDER (ADHD)

"Candy corn is not a vegetable."
—AUTHOR UNKNOWN

Attention-deficit hyperactivity disorder (ADHD) has been clouded in controversy since the 1970s. Many have wondered about the authenticity of this nebulous disorder, cast doubt on the accuracy of its diagnosis, and questioned the use of stimulants (particularly the widespread use of Ritalin) in children. We certainly feel strongly that safer alternative approaches should be tried before subjecting children to any drug regimen.

THE STANDARD DEFINITION OF ADHD

ADHD is considered a neurobehavioral developmental disorder of children that is characterized by difficulty staying focused and paying attention, out-of-control behavior, and over-activity. It is thought to affect 3–5 percent of children worldwide, but is actually diagnosed in 2–16 percent of school-aged children (at least twice as often in boys than girls).[1] However, even the American Academy of Pediatrics acknowledges that these figures could be inaccurate: "Recorded prevalence rates for ADHD vary substantially, partly because of changing diagnostic criteria over time, and partly because of variations in ascertainment in different settings and the frequent use of referred samples to estimate rates. Practitioners of all types (primary care, subspecialty, psychiatry, and non-physician mental health providers) vary greatly in the degree in which they use *Diagnostic and Statistical Manual of Mental Health Disorders Fourth Edition* (DSM-IV) criteria to diagnose ADHD. Reported rates also vary substantially in different geographic areas and across countries."[2]

There are three basic subtypes of ADHD, according to the DSM-IV: predominantly inattentive, predominantly hyperactive-impulsive, and combined hyperactive-impulsive and inattentive.[3]

Symptoms of those predominantly inattentive:

- Easily distracted, miss details, forget things

- Difficulty maintaining focus

- Easily become bored

- Don't listen when spoken to

- Prone to daydreaming, easily confused

- Do not follow instructions

Symptoms of those predominantly hyperactive-impulsive:

- Fidgeting and squirming

- Nonstop talking

- Tendency to run around, touching everything in sight

- Difficulty participating in quiet activities

Symptoms of those with the combined type also include:

- Extreme impatience

- Tendency to make inappropriate comments, be overly emotional, and act out without regard for others[4]

While it is normal for all children to be inattentive, hyperactive, or impulsive at times, these behaviors are present to a more severe degree and occur more often in those with ADHD, according to the conventional definition of the disorder. To be diagnosed, children must exhibit symptoms in two different settings, such as at school and at home, for at least six months and to a more exaggerated degree than seen in other children.

Conventional medicine experts admit that the cause of ADHD is unknown,[5] even after decades of research. A number of factors are thought to contribute to the condition, including a potential genetic link, environmental factors (tobacco smoke; complications or infections during the mother's pregnancy; exposure to insecticides, lead, and pesticides), and diet (particularly food colorings).

Common treatments used for ADHD include stimulant (Ritalin) and nonstimulant (atomoxetine) medications and behavioral and psychological therapies.

A CONTROVERSIAL HISTORY

The attention-deficit syndrome developed in the late 1950s. Many cultural changes were just getting underway at that time. Mothers became more "busy," so *all* time was no longer *quality* time. TV watching, with all its hype, discouraged the increase in attention span that quiet reading on mother's lap provided to the preschooler, as well as displacing time for motherly guidance. The "baby boomers" were, by their sheer numbers, overwhelming pediatricians' offices, causing the physicians to cut down on the time needed to know their patients, time needed to solve problems and to educate. It was the beginning of "patch 'em up" medicine in lieu of preventive medicine. The food industry was developing and promoting processed foods that were attractive, had a long shelf-life, and would sell, by adding generous amounts of sugar, food coloring, and anything else—nutrient deficient or not—that would appeal to the shopper. Last but not least, child psychologists and psychiatrists were coming out of the woodwork with all kinds of excuses for bad behavior in school.

A syndrome consists of a collection of signs (objective findings, seen by the observer) and symptoms (subjective findings, described by the patient) that are presumed to appear, more or less consistently, in different patients affected by the same causal factors. If the causal factors can be consistently identified, a diagnosis can be attached to the patient. If causal factors are more ambiguous, not to worry—the patient can probably still fit into one syndrome or the other. And there is some room for forgiveness if the criteria almost fit, but not quite.

ADHD was previously known by many names, including: attention-deficit disorder, minimal brain dysfunction in children, hyperkinetic child syndrome, minimal brain damage, and minor cerebral dysfunction. The use of these diagnostic labels leaves us asking, "How can my child, who must have something wrong with his brain, be blamed for his behavior?" With such an ominous diagnosis as this (just look at all those medical words), one could easily think, "I certainly hope there is a treatment. I am so glad to have found that the way I have raised him has nothing to do with his behavior. As far as my responsibilities as a parent go, in this particular matter, I am off the hook."

A child who showed strong opposition to his or her parent's orders was given the diagnosis of "oppositional-defiant disorder" by psychiatrists. This could be considered as "co-morbid" with ADHD. One wonders if these disorders might be more readily accepted if more honestly renamed to "obnoxious brat disorder" or "holy terror disorder." Of course, there is no attempt to claim that the stimulant medication will treat the associated disorder, but there is a strong implication that by treating ADHD, the associated disorders might be less apparent.

The early descriptions of the syndrome put more emphasis on the inability to sit still. Later, it was decided that this hyperactivity was due to the child's inability to pay attention, and he had to do something, so the emphasis shifted to this lack of concentration. Making "boredom" a precursor of the problem does not sound as scientific as "the inability of the limbic system to filter out unnecessary stimuli."

Some clinicians are uncomfortable accepting a syndrome that has no known cause. The *Physicians' Desk Reference* (PDR) states, "Specific etiology for this syndrome is unknown." Do any of these diagnoses supply a hint as to their cause or what we might do about it if we do find a cause? Also, some are concerned about the pressure to treat with a medication whose mode of action is unclear. Says the PDR: "The mode of action in man is not completely understood, but Ritalin *presumably* activates the brainstem arousal system and cortex to support its stimulant effect."

One 2001 survey found that ADHD is "due to developmental and genetic factors that affect biochemical and metabolic function."[6] What function of mind or body is not due to biochemical factors, determined by our DNA? Again, statements like this are designed only to provide a sense of scientific legitimacy. They give the unbelievable figure of "30–40 percent of children with ADHD have relatives with this disorder." They did lower the estimate of the percentage of the school-age population with this disorder to 3–5 percent. The survey was based on 255 children with the disorder and 252 without. They concluded that about a quarter with ADHD have problems participating in after-school activities. Of course, if the diagnosis includes anti-social behavior, who wants to play with these kids? Less than a quarter participate in behavioral therapy. How many can afford it? Also, 89 percent were prescribed medications, but only 55 percent of these take them and those who do tend to not take the drugs on the weekends. Does this tell us that the problem is a problem only in school? If the medication were truly helpful, I think parents would welcome the improvement when their child is around them.

According to the PDR, "Ritalin is indicated as an integral part of a total treatment program which typically includes other remedial measures (psychological, educational, social) for a stabilizing effect in children with a behavioral syndrome characterized by the following group of developmentally inappropriate symptoms: moderate-to-severe distractibility, short attention span, hyperactivity, emotional lability and impulsivity." This is followed by the admonition: "The diagnosis of this syndrome should not be made with finality when these symptoms are only of comparatively recent origin. Soft neurological signs, learning disabilities, and abnormal EEG *may or may not* be present, and a diagnosis *may or may not* be present." How's that for backtracking?

No Specific Diagnosis

The compulsion to reduce everything to statistics in order to lend support to a hypothesis seems to be a modern-day hang-up of medical "scientists." In listing diagnostic criteria for ADHD, the behavior in question is preceded by the word *often*. The question becomes, "How often is often?" If we are going to get picky with figures, shouldn't we be able to pick a figure of how many times per unit of time? It is counterproductive to attempt to make precise diagnoses with such subjective material.

Since we don't know the specific cause, there is no specific diagnostic test. Input from psychologists, educators, and social workers is needed in addition to medical input. Stimulants are not recommended for those with more defined causes, such as environmental factors (could this include diet?), psychiatric disorders, even psychosis. "Appropriate educational placement is essential, and psychosocial intervention is generally necessary. When remedial measures alone are insufficient, the decision to prescribe stimulant medication will depend upon the physician's assessment of the chronicity and severity of the child's symptoms." Unfortunately, this tedious protocol is not followed by prescribing physicians. Ritalin prescriptions are handed out all too freely.

When Proctor & Gamble comes out with "New, Improved Blue Cheer," the box is different and the blue color of the detergent is new, but basically it is the same stuff that used to get your clothes clean. Ciba, the pharmaceutical company that produces Ritalin, is in the marketing business and knows these marketing techniques. The new and improved medical lingo lent to this syndrome provides an aura of knowing their stuff. In the early 1960s, before I was on to them, I conscientiously studied and attended conferences at which I would learn of this syndrome and of the "soft neurological signs" that were supposed to be a reflection of some kind of brain damage. I laugh as I recall patient and doctor sitting opposite each other and seeing how fast each could alternately slap his respective knees with the palms and then the backs of their hands. Then, we would see how fast the patient could touch the index fingers of the outstretched hands of the physician with his own index fingers. The testing was completed with touching of the respective noses with alternate index fingers. Speed was the key, and the physician's speed was the gold standard. If the patient flunked, the ominous word *dyskinesia* was entered into his chart.

Soon, school psychologists were devising their own tests for dyskinesia and instructing teachers in the art of mass screening. One gangly third grader failed to stand on his desk on only one leg, like the rest of his classmates, and was referred to me. He proved to be a bit awkward, but nothing out of line considering his height, build, and immaturity. I concluded my exam as a figure, who proved to be his father, lumbered in from the waiting room. He was a large man and certainly had the biggest feet I ever saw. As necessary as they were for support of this big man, they seemed to function independently of the rest of him. Do you think I was going to tell him that his son was clumsy and that my medical education was so deficient that I could not understand how he got that way? Neither could I be honest and apologize for the blunders of the ignorant school staff, even though they were well intentioned.

Later, these same counselors were asking parents if their kids had ever had a high fever or if they knew of any gross errors the obstetrician had made during delivery. Ritalin treatment was thoroughly embraced by some, as Ciba's attempts at verification seemed more and more "scientific." Ciba has achieved with Ritalin what only one other stimulant, caffeine, has achieved—worldwide acceptance. What is a stimulant? It stimulates the brain as well as other organs, such as the heart. Lack of attention or lack of concentration should be helped by that effect. There is now a question of how much improvement in cognition there is from a cup of coffee, since the effect may just be alleviation of the worsened intellectual abilities brought about from the initial withdrawal. I will concede the point that a stimulant should help when there is poor concentration, but it might help for whatever the reason concentration is poor.

There was not another medication in the PDR whose suggested use is in conjunction with "psychological, educational, and social resources." (Look-alike medications appeared later on.) Support for the use of Ritalin cannot come from medical doctors alone—it must include believers from the ranks of school psychologists, educators, and social workers as well. Ciba sponsors "support groups" of parents of kids with this syndrome, attended by pediatric neurologists, general psychiatrists, doctors of various descriptions (including pediatricians), school psychologists, teachers, and social workers. I am embarrassed to see members of my profession attend these sessions.

Is Ritalin the Answer?

In 1994, I received a letter from Mrs. Sally Brunday of the United Kingdom. She wrote as follows: "It seems that the U.K. is now being swamped with literature on the wonders of Ritalin for ADHD and dyslexic children. We (our organization, The Hyperactive Children's Support Group, for hyperactive, allergic and learning-disabled children) have been in existence for seventeen years and are determined to fight the drug onslaught and continue our efforts through dietary nutritional means, for the sake of the children." She requested any "materials/evidence that we can present to the dyslexia groups and others to support our case against these drugs."

I wrote this in response to her request:

> It represents what I had learned from seeing many children suspected of suffering from this disorder.
>
> I am happy to see some media attention being brought to bear on the nearly thoughtless use of Ritalin. Just the description of the drug in the Physicians' Desk Reference appears to suggest that it is a drug of low self-esteem that has, for thirty-five years, been trying to feel useful; or to give the appearance, at least, that it is useful. Ciba Pharmaceuticals, the manufacturer, has attempted to tie Ritalin's usefulness to the treatment of nebulous psycho-neurological diseases (or disorders) and one more tangible disorder (narcolepsy). To lend scientific authenticity to this link, the description of the syndrome that Ritalin is to treat is very ambiguous, fraught with a name change every few years, and it involves lots of medical terms that even we physicians in the trenches have to look up.
>
> The PDR states that "Ritalin is a mild central nervous system stimulant." (Amphetamines are stimulants also, but not to worry.)

That, by definition, means it increases wakefulness. The other indication for the drug is for the treatment of narcolepsy, a rare syndrome of untoward sleepiness. A student dozing off during a lecture might show the low end of the spectrum of narcolepsy. Ritalin possibly could be the appropriate treatment if a less problematic cup of coffee failed to correct this behavior. The top end of narcolepsy is the more serious condition of suddenly going "out," usually requiring treatment with a stronger amphetamine derivative.

The PDR requires the contributing company to post all adverse reactions. Ritalin is no exception. "In children, loss of appetite, abdominal pain, weight loss during prolonged therapy, insomnia, and tachycardia, may occur more frequently. . . . Nervousness and insomnia are the most common adverse reactions." But the indicated remedy is to simply reduce the dose. The laundry list of severe and very serious medical problems is scary. It includes several life-threatening conditions, psychological abnormalities such as Tourette's syndrome, acute psychosis, and transient depression, as well as headaches and drowsiness. Dyskinesia is mentioned as a side effect of Ritalin—strange, in that dyskinesia was a diagnostic "soft sign," a marker for the syndrome that should be managed with this drug. Remember that dyskinesia is a fancy name for being poorly coordinated. But "serious" dyskinesia refers to a drug reaction that causes tics or muscle spasm of the neck and facial muscles.

Finally, why is a significant part of society that is concerned about drug usage and desires drug-free buildings (including schools) spreading the word of the wonders of Ritalin and paying a school nurse to dispense it? Is it because of the belief that Ritalin might make a kid behave better or at least make him more manageable in the classroom? What kind of hypocrisy is this? There are documented incidents of kids on prescribed Ritalin who have had it foisted on them, who do not like this drug, but are happy to sell it to someone who thinks he can get high on any illicit substance.

ALTERNATIVE TREATMENTS FOR ADHD

Clearly, I (RC) do not like drug treatment for this behavior syndrome.

Unfortunately, the longer the problem persists without the benefit of non-pharmaceutical intervention, the more difficult it is to reverse the faulty behavior. While getting on track with nutrition advice, strong effort has to be made to achieve acceptable behavior at school and at home.

In my earlier years, after moving to Montana, my way of diagnosis and treatment was well accepted by the school system. I had many patient referrals directly from school personnel or indirectly from "word of mouth." I would explain the "crazy" concept that a food allergen could affect the nervous system so as to produce this behavioral problem. However, I had to be careful when speaking of "brain allergy" when the parent and I were not on the same page. After I obtained a careful medical history and a completed a thorough, appropriate physical examination, I explained to the parents how to try the "detection-and-challenge" method of identifying food allergens. Even though dramatic improvement often came after the offending allergens were removed, offensive behavioral patterns that had become habituated still needed to be changed.

The term *developmentally inappropriate behavior* is quite inventive. When it is defined as distractibility, short attention span, hyperactivity, emotional lability (instability), and impulsivity, it reminds us that generic two-year-olds usually exhibit all of the above; however, it is inappropriate to retain these behavior patterns until school age. I can't give parents a diagnosis that will get them completely off the hook for failure to make developmental progress. Increase of attention span is a process, and sitting still is a learned thing one has to practice. With parental guidance and perseverance, much emotional instability is overcome, and it can always be tempered; it needs to be overcome by the time a young person is turned loose on society.

If parents realize what I just stated but believe progress is too slow, a general pediatric evaluation should be done. Even Ciba agrees that a thoughtful diagnosis should be made before prescribing Ritalin. I will rarely (almost never) prescribe Ritalin. I would ask questions about early child rearing, older siblings, and any family history of this type of behavior. If there was another family member with a similar problem, when did they grow out of it? Has this child shown any allergies in the past? If so, what kind and to what? Of course, what I mean by "allergy" may not be what they mean; I would point out how certain allergies can affect behavior. I would also ask if the child is often on an even keel but has "Jekyll and Hyde–like" outbursts when his behavior is simply horrid.

Altering Behavior

If your child exhibits more mental and physical energy than average, there is a good chance a health professional or some authoritative voice from his school is going to suggest that he suffers from ADHD. The more he weighs in on the energy scale, the more demanding is the need to "do something." The first something should be to arrange for a conference between you, the parent, and whoever made the "tentative diagnosis." Even the pharmaceutical companies who make the drugs designed to control behavior associated with this disorder state that a complete medical evaluation is needed. The main purpose of evaluation is to define the parameters of normal behavior and see where the lines are crossed. Before medical treatment is even remotely considered, a parent should not be afraid to ask about alternative ways of addressing this "problem." Beware of a push for medication before taking these steps.

Look at the *individuality* of your infant or child, not as one put into a general, drug-treated diagnostic category. Decide, by your own sense of what is normal, if your child fits into an accepted range of normal. Check with friends whose judgment you trust to see if their observations agree with yours. If school authorities or other professionals suggest your child's behavior exceeds the range of normal and should be treated for ADHD, ask for specific reasons for their determination. If his behavior is disrupting, this will need to be modified. If there are outbursts of behavior in the morning, see if this behavior is replicated under your observation at home. If so, look for a food allergen or hypoglycemia reaction.

Feel confident that you can manage without drugs. "Just say no!" If you are urged to subject your child to drug therapy, have your health professional review the PDR description of the drug, including the drawbacks.

Let us consider the challenge of raising an *active* child, let alone a hyperactive child, with or without a diagnostic label. A new mom can appreciate a "good" baby who seemingly is content with little more than a full tummy and uninterrupted sleep. On the other hand, there is the super-active infant that was "shot out of a cannon": he may be fully aware of things around him and doesn't want to miss a single drumbeat of life. True, mother gets more sleep with the quiet type, while raising the active child is much more work. There are medical conditions that create either type, but basically differentiation is seen in the newborn, much the same as in a litter of pups. Which pup do we select? Do we want the quiet one or the one full of life? Both may be highly intelligent, but the curious mind is easier to observe. The child-rearing task is to encourage and stimulate the more passive one and respect the potential for toning down the active one without stifling his personality. What is it that the ADHD drugs are attempting to control?

Offensive behavior patterns must be identified and freely discussed, and a good deal of parental support is needed. Before a child is able to think things through and understand that his actions affect not only his life but also the lives around him, he has to depend on parents to consistently set standards of acceptable behavior. Experts say that abstract thinking doesn't appear until age eight, but habits of behavior need to be established far in advance of this. Ordinary, "wise" suggestions for child rearing, presented in a way that will neither insult intelligence nor elicit guilt feelings, often help. It is surprising how a very ordinary suggestion can be quite profound when it is something the parent always knew but had forgotten to consider. Never would I suggest a trial of medication before a trial of appropriate changes in diet or the application of common sense, consistent measures for the specific undesirable behavior. If attention span is short, lengthen it. If he can't sit still, give age-appropriate things to do with the hands, during which time the rest of the body is still. Play games where he is encouraged to *not* sit still but to concentrate (for example, "Keep your eyes on the ball"). Many of these remedies require parental input for which a medication cannot substitute.

Inability to pay attention in the classroom may simply be due to boredom and lack of challenge of an active, keen mind. Top-notch enriched or special education can accomplish wonders for these children. Hyperactivity, as defined in this syndrome, is similar. We fidget when bored, but doodling or other patterns of inattentiveness have no place in the classroom. Uncontrollable outbursts that disrupt the classroom, and can be associated with legitimate psychiatric disorders, can be related to food allergies and the "wooly-brained" or "spacey" condition that results. Or, being "uncontrollable" can exist from a fixed pattern of never having been subjected to appropriate parental control. Symptom relief with medication is not sufficient—underlying causes must be explored and dealt with.

Keep challenging an active mind and supplementing your child's schoolwork. Perhaps there would be a need for his reading aloud at home or for getting help in the selection of suitable reading material. If your child has too much physical energy, find an activity that will constructively use some of the excess. Besides the health benefit, gaining athletic prowess won't hurt a bit in gaining acceptance. In addition, a degree of self-control is needed. When a child feels that he is losing control of his behavior, he should make a special effort to be "nice" and think of what the teacher and his fellow students would expect from him.

Changing the Diet

Sugar Allergy and Hypoglycemia

Sugar is a common cause of disruptive outbursts when it acts as an allergen or a precipitator of low blood sugar, which leads to subsequent adrenaline and norepinephrine release, stimulating hormones that cause sympathetic nervous system signs. Maybe we do not know how Ritalin functions, but we do know a lot about cerebral dysfunction that results from a drop in blood glucose. Since the brain must have glucose for fuel, there are many safety checks in place to prevent brain damage. When the blood glucose level reaches a high level too quickly, after eating a sweet (or refined starch), too much insulin is called into play. Two or three hours later, when hypoglycemia results, adrenaline is brought into action in order to release more glucose into the bloodstream from muscle tissue and the liver. This is a safety mechanism to prevent the brain from being deprived of glucose.

In the medical literature, the commonality of hypoglycemia signs and symptoms in children and ADHD behavior appeared in the early 1990s.[7] After a glucose-loading test, children showed late postprandial (after ingestion) levels of epinephrine (adrenaline) at twice the level of adults and were more apt to be sweaty and feel shaky. The children's glucose levels did not have to fall as far as an adult's to create the epinephrine response. Thus, children are more vulnerable to the effects of hypoglycemia on cognitive function than adults, because the drop in glucose that sets off the epinephrine response is more modest and is mediated through the nervous system (norepinephrine). Other research related aggressive behavior to low serotonin in those who show hypoglycemia in a glucose tolerance test.[8] There are numerous other studies correlating aggressive behavior to hypoglycemia. It is strange that hypoglycemia is so common, yet the connection of behavior problems and hypoglycemia is seldom recognized.

Conventional researchers have long tried to put to bury the idea that sugar has anything to do with the etiology of ADHD. They say that double-blind studies in nutrition cannot achieve meaningful results because of "confounding variables," including deficiencies of vitamins that act as cofactors in the formation of neurotransmitters, interaction with other nutrients, wide individual differences, and any number of enzymatic reactions. A million kindergarten teachers can't be wrong as they speculate that the behavior they see on November 1st is the result of a sugar hangover from the famous evening before.

The scientific proof of sensitivity or allergy to sugar or other food ingredients is a three-step process.

1. Suspect—Note signs and symptoms that may indicate a sensitivity or allergy after the child has had anything to eat or drink.

2. Eliminate—Remove the suspected allergen completely from the diet for several days and note loss of the signs and symptoms.

3. Challenge—If not absolutely sure, challenge with the suspected allergen. If you are correct, the signs and symptoms will return.

FOOD ADDITIVES AND CHILDREN'S BEHAVIOR

Allergist Benjamin Feingold, M.D., was one of the first physicians to speak out against food additives. His special concerns were the effect of food chemicals on children's behavior and the role of nutrition in treating learning disabilities. The chemical food processing industry, and its pseudo-scientific spokespersons, are still trying to negate Feingold's research. It will never happen, though, because Feingold Associations of informed parents (and forward-thinking doctors) are to found worldwide.

Children's learning and behavior problems often begin in our grocery cart. Says the Feingold Association: "Numerous studies show that certain synthetic food additives can have serious learning, behavior, and/or health effects for sensitive people." Dr. Feingold's diet eliminated food additives, especially food dyes. He felt there was a strong correlation between these artificial ingredients and ADHD. In a nutrition study, it is difficult to zero in on the effect of just one ingredient, since a food consists of many influencing factors. Food additives are usually mingled with sugar, and we feel sugar is a prime suspect.[9]

Recent evidence published in the *Lancet*[10] confirms the validity of Dr. Feingold's approach. A rigorous randomized, double-blind, placebo-controlled crossover study of nearly 300 children showed "significantly adverse effect compared with placebo" when they consumed artificial colors and/or the preservative sodium benzoate. These additives specifically resulted in increased hyperactivity.

Sometimes, I will prescribe extra B vitamins (a B-50 supplement with breakfast), especially pyridoxine (B_6; 100 mg with another meal) and magnesium (200–250 mg), or other specific dietary suggestions, depending on what we have learned in the history.

Healthier Eating

A solid breakfast is a must. This is the time to fuel up for the day ahead, so provide more slow-burning protein and little or no refined carbohydrates. This also is a good time to include fat in order to avoid midmorning low blood sugar with the resulting hunger and inability to concentrate.

Breakfast should be preceded by a good night's sleep. There are no rigid rules, but ten hours for a youngster in the early grades usually is the norm. Individual differences in requirement can be measured by observing whether your child is raring to go or is barely awake after making his way to the breakfast table. Gaining regularity in sleep patterns, as in eating patterns, is very helpful—not something rigidly controlled, but patterns that promote predictability.

A COLORFUL SALUTE TO VALENTINE'S DAY

Those little candy hearts with "I LUV U" and "BE MINE" imprinted on them have a special secret—they make great children's paints! I (AWS) like to try this with kids: have them collect their candy hearts, especially the purple ones, grind them up, combine equal parts water and powdered candy, and stir. Get out a model-sized paintbrush and white paper and have the children write their names in food paint. It works all too well. Then, ask the kids what it does to their stomachs. Listen carefully to their answers and insights.

When I taught junior high school, I wondered where the girls' rather weird-colored hairdos came from. The girls 'fessed up: they dyed their hair with "Kool Aid." This is not a new idea, it turns out. In the film *The Wizard of Oz*, the animals used as the Horse of a Different Color were colored, from fetlock to mane, with a mixture of "Jell-O" powder.

I concede that artificial colors are great for dying horses' hair and painting pictures, but I am not convinced that we should voluntarily eat paint. So read every label and vote with your dollars. Then send the only message that carries any weight in the food industry: *do not purchase any food that contains an artificial food coloring.*

In order to establish life-long health habits, explain to your child how vitamins and diet help. Have him think about what makes him feel out of sorts and tell you about it. Get to the point to where he, on his own volition, asks for his vitamins every morning.

The neurotransmitters norepinephrine and serotonin are in a see-saw relationship—if one is up, the other is down. Balance is achieved not by a drug that acts to either suppress or enhance one or the other, but in supplying the means for making the neurotransmitters as they are needed. For a school-aged child, provide vitamin C in the form of 500 mg tasty chewtabs, given in divided doses (mealtimes), one or two at a time. In order to avoid a hassle at school lunchtime, provide two tabs at breakfast. A B-50 preparation will provide the necessary niacin (B_3) and pyridoxine (B_6).

If a smooth behavior pattern has not been achieved after a sufficient trial, work on either adding more omega-3 fatty acids (fish oils) to the diet or getting a better omega-3 to omega-6 fatty acid ratio. Do this by reducing the omega-6s (the vegetable oils) while at the same time strictly avoiding trans-fat intake (hydrogenated vegetable oils). Check your food labels. For example, mayonnaise comes in several forms: the cheap vegetable oil source (such as soybean oil), or canola or olive oil, both of which are monounsaturated fatty acids superior to omega-6 fatty acids. This is not a quick fix but a long-term help, as these fatty acids eventually end up in every cell membrane, including those of the nervous system. Besides aiding nervous system function, there are many other health benefits derived from reducing the formation of inflammation promoters.

The next chapter will provide some additional suggestions for changing problem behavior in children without the use of drugs.

SUMMARY

These children are not dull, but they are challenging. We desire active citizens in our society. Our aim is to channel the positives and gradually do away with the negatives early in life. Drug-induced behavioral control, by diminishing positive personality traits along with negative traits, should not be the solution. The question is, how do we define hyperactivity? Too much of a good thing or too much of a bad thing? Take advice from the old Harold Arlen/Johnny Mercer tune "Ac-Cent-Tchu-Ate the Positive":

You've got to accentuate the positive

Eliminate the negative

And enjoy observing the evolution of a great kid. After getting at the nutritional basis and after great strides have been made in achieving acceptable behavior, this positive personality demands a lot of parental guidance. It is important, and you can do it!

CHAPTER 11

HOW TO IMPROVE
A CHILD'S BEHAVIOR
WITHOUT DRUGS

*"Not only is example the best way to teach,
it is the only way."*
—ALBERT SCHWEITZER, M.D.

We are concerned about the lack of "bringing up" children today, from the standpoint of both pediatricians and the parents. It is a "no no," and just plain unhelpful, to lecture about acceptable standards of behavior unless that is what the individual parent wants. But we see a very important spin-off of establishing standards of behavior early in life: eating habits and taking vitamin supplements become as automatic and acceptable to children as brushing teeth. The earlier parents take charge, the less likelihood of a moody or rebellious school-aged child.

CHILD BEHAVIOR MANAGEMENT

If there were a genuine shortcut to raising children, kids would be ready to go off on their own by age two. If this concept appeals to you, I (AWS) recommend that you change species, for a two-year-old cat, dog, or cow is fully adult. Whales, elephants, and humans seem to take a rather long time to mature. Given that your offspring are not *really* the animals they sometimes appear to be, and that they are therefore going to be hanging about for some time, here are some techniques that may prove useful in the everyday trenches of childrea-ring. We will start with the emergency procedure first.

Niacin

This is not in any of the how-to-raise-kids books that I've ever seen, but it's extremely important. Give niacin (vitamin B_3) to fussy children and fussy teenagers. How much? Just enough to barely "flush" them. This nearly inevitable (and harmless) "hot flash" experience indicates saturation of niacin. When a child is at niacin saturation, they are biochemically mellowed inside. Niacin is the preeminent natural, safe, cheap, all-purpose antidepressant/anti-anxiety/antipsychotic vitamin.

If you still think that discipline is the only way to handle kids in difficult situations (or difficult kids in normal situations), you are missing out on a wonderful opportunity. Try some niacin, starting with about 25 milligrams per dose, with doses every 10 minutes until the child cools off (or, rather, gets warm). If the child does not want to take it, these steps may help: take some niacin yourself (about 50–100 mg) right in front of the child. Not only does this set a good example, it is also fair, and it will calm you down as well. That will make the entire situation less volatile.

Dr. Campbell found a modest-dose B-complex supplement (50 mg of most B vitamins) helpful in keeping a child on a more even keel after correcting the basic physical causes first (much like we described in the previous chapter). The high-dose niacin treatment could work well for stopping a real outburst. As with any behavioral problem, the child needs to understand why his or her behavior is inappropriate and that correction is not entirely a passive affair. The child will need to try to do better. The following method may help bring this about.

1-2-3 Count

Time honored but somehow still largely unknown, master teachers and expert parents have been using this system for decades. My mom (a history teacher during World War Two) used this on my brothers and me back in the 1950s. She also tried other, less effective methods, as we all have. Too bad, for this technique alone, consistently performed, is entirely adequate and utterly nonviolent.

It works like this: tell your child that you are going to give them three strikes before they are "out" and sent to their room for fifteen minutes. The first time your child says or does anything you do not want her to, say "one." The very next time it happens, say "two." The third time, say "three" (or "take fifteen" or "time out," whatever suits you). At this, the child is to go directly to her room and must stay in her room for the duration of the penalty. It's just like in a hockey game, but "count" them before any teeth are missing. A good rule of thumb is ten minutes for a little kid, fifteen minutes for a preteen, and twenty minutes for a teenager. (No use of electronic gadgets allowed during time out.)

Initially, you may have to take the child to her room and endure the howls of misery and injustice. Just shut the door, set a kitchen timer, and leave. If the child comes out, take her back in and restart the timer. If you feel that you are having a really tough time with your child, I recommend reading *1, 2, 3 Magic* by Thomas Phelan, Ph.D.[1] Better yet, watch his video of the same title. It is extremely well done, and I think you might see your child, so to speak, in the many examples shown.

Parent, Know Thyself

My shorthand kid-management system is basically this:

- Decide what you want
- Make it clear to all concerned
- See that you get it
- Put a time on it
- Put a consequence on it

"Deciding what you want" is more important than it sounds. For years, I have told students that if you do not understand the question, you cannot possibly get the right answer. If adults do not know what really matters to them personally, they have little hope of achieving fulfillment. Sample starter questions to spur your thinking: If money were no object, what would you do with your life? What always makes you happy? Who do you most admire, and why? If you had three wishes, what would they be? What do you think about before going to sleep? What's first on your mind when you awake? What did you never have that you want your children to have? I'll bet you can quickly add to this list.

"Making it clear to all concerned" stops an age-old communication problem dead in its tracks. Do not wait to be asked—express a need in simple, unambiguous terms. Then, be prepared to listen for the other person's needs too. Tactical hint: for best results, reverse these steps. Listen first, and restate what the other person has said to show them they have been understood, then state your needs to a now much more receptive set of ears. It is probably best to limit this to two or three of your needs at a time. Pick the ones you cannot live without right up front.

"See that you get it." Be honest with yourself: are you on the path toward your bliss, your most heartfelt goals? Are you in a relationship that enlivens your life? Is there a better job for you? For parents, asking yourself, "What single action can I take today to enrich my life?" can also be surprisingly productive, especially after you see that one goal met per day is thirty goals in only a month. And specifically with regard to raising children, be consistent. In the film *The Last Emperor,* the tutor to the young emperor told him, "If you do not say what you mean, you will never mean what you say." Do you mean what you say? When I was a student teacher, my excellent mentor, Hugh Ratigan, Ed.D, taught me early on that follow-through is the big one. If you say it, you have to do it. To avoid this dilemma, shut up. I cannot tell you how many times I found Mark Twain's advice to be right on the money, especially: "It is better to remain silent and be thought a fool than to speak and remove all doubt." If you make a rule, you have to enforce it. My personal solution to this has been to keep the rules to very few. Only the important stuff deserves your enforcement. Having had thirty-seven teenagers in a chemistry laboratory, I am here to tell you that safety and cooperation rules are essential.

"Put a time on it" to help you focus on the present and "be here now." That timer technique, mentioned above, is part of it for the kids. Time limits on telephone and television are reasonable and appropriate. I feel that making sure children are home at a specific time is very important. We had a clipboard by the front door for signing out and in. This is not tyrannical, for it only takes a minute for a kid to put their initials, their destination, and a friend's name or phone number down on a notepad. My son, even as a teenager, said that he would definitely do this with his own kids. That may be the highest form of praise.

"Put a consequence on it." Consequences that work all share one common feature—they are nonviolent. Spanking and hitting simply do not work. Time-outs, fines on allowances, and suspending TV privileges all work. Or let the children themselves devise their own negative consequences. This, by the way, is one of the oldest and sneakiest teacher tricks in the book: let the kids make the consequences. You will be surprised by how strict they can be with themselves.

Do not forget positive consequences. One of my favorite aphorisms is "Really surprise someone today: catch them doing something right." Kids of all ages love praise. I learned this, of all places, from viewing "Mister Rogers' Neighborhood." I even used it when I taught at two state penitentiaries. It worked, of course. Fred Rogers reinforced how true it is that people of all ages respond to praise. Kids will work hard for a teacher's approval, the smiles as much as the grades. Adults will work hard for a spouse's approval. It is a bit hard to fathom it at times, but your own children work harder if you can give them approval, too. I suggest the following: promptly reward good behavior in a tangible way. Gifts, favorite activities, spending money, a meal out, parent-made "coupons" for special privileges, and other child- and teen-pleasers are worth using from time to time. Remember that there is a real need for parent "teacher" and the child "student" to constantly work together toward improvement.

It's important to note, however, that you should avoid rewarding a child's good behavior with tokens like candies simply for the sake of building "self esteem." Most children see through a phony deal. What they seek is genuine praise, administered with love. When they behave well and receive praise, they automatically feel good about themselves. The association of reward with sweets is not a healthy one.

DAILY PRIORITIES IN LIFE

When I (AWS) was a boy, my father and mother told me that I could not go far wrong if I followed these guidelines:

- Your health first
- Your family second
- Your job (or, for kids, your schoolwork) third

I figured out myself that everything else is fourth. (As a now-experienced parent, I am persuaded to add this to this list "TV and video games last!")

Health includes getting plenty of sleep, eating proper meals, getting exercise, taking appropriate amounts of vitamin supplements, and using an organized system of relaxation and self-improvement, such as meditation or prayer. These are life's first duties. You are obligated to take care of your soul and body in order to do anything else, so your health is number one.

Family is in second place, only second because if you are not healthy and well rested, you cannot be at your best as a spouse or a parent. "Family" may be divided into two priorities: your spouse first, and the children follow a close but definite second. It is important for all, especially kids, to understand that mom and dad loved each other first, and children came along next. Children exist because of a couple's initial love for each other, so the couple must therefore have the higher priority. A happy couple will be an automatic benefit to the children. The marriage relationship needs to come first. There are enough divorces to show that too often it doesn't.

Job or schoolwork takes third place. This can be of profound help to harried breadwinners and anxious students. Most of us have been, or will be, both. As a kid, it helped me to know that staying up very late to do homework was not the answer. It was also not permitted by my parents. If we were exhausted, the homework did not get done. If we put it off until the last minute, we had a problem. I'd like to say that my brothers and I therefore never put off homework, but that isn't true. What we did learn was that it was wise to begin our homework early. In college, I'd head for the library right after my last class and do as much studying before supper as possible. Right after supper, it was back to the library. By about 8 P.M. or so, I was walking out of the library when most everyone else was walking in. I was done, with the evening free before me, while they hadn't even begun.

The day my daughter was born, there was a big event at work lasting from noon until almost midnight. It was important financially and had been long planned in advance. At 9 A.M., I was at the hospital with my one-hour old baby girl. I checked the priority list: I picked family over job, did not go to work that day, and lost money. I've frequently looked back on that decision with no regrets. Every time I see my daughter, I know I had my priorities straight. It was only one day, but it means a lot to me now. The company that I then worked for has since gone out of business.

CORRECTION INSTITUTIONS OR CORRECTIVE NUTRITION?

Many years ago, during teacher training, we were taught that we would graduate more criminals than scientists. A sobering thought to be sure. But what happens, ultimately, if behavior or poor nutrition is uncorrected? We think the two are closely related. Dr. Campbell was a jail doctor, and I (AWS) used to teach college courses in two state penitentiaries. We have both seen a part of life that, we fervently hope, you and your children never will.

Let us give it to you straight: prisons are awful places. First of all, they smell, and you still have the fundamental and repugnant problem of packing as many as possible into the space available. The "keep the lid on the garbage can" theory serves the public to be sure, but there are more Americans incarcerated per capita than in any other Western country. After all, the argument goes, what do we care about their living conditions? They get three square meals a day, clean sheets, and a roof over their head for free. With some 2.4 million Americans behind bars, serious overcrowding continues. The state is doing us a real favor putting most of these characters away.

The most frightening man I have ever seen was not on a movie or TV screen. He was an inmate at the medium-security prison where I was teaching in 1991. Like most of my students (I called them my "captive audience"), he really didn't belong in a college science class. Not that he, or the others, were a discipline problem, because they usually weren't. He had simply never had a single high school science class, the most basic prerequisite for even my simplified, freshman-level biology course.

So, this big guy struggled with the material, nose down to his book, week after week. It occasionally crossed my mind that it might be good for the whole inmate population if this man passed the course; it might be good for *me* too.

During one class, I was lecturing on human nutrition and mentioned foods that are especially wholesome, such as beans, whole-grain bread, wheat germ, and so on. To spark class interest, I asked what foods the prisoners were fed. White bread, meat, potatoes, and sugar was the general consensus.

"What about vitamin supplements?" I asked.

This really got them going. "No, they never give 'em to us," came the reply. "Got to buy them yourself at the commissary store. They only have 'One-a-Day' multiple vitamin pills there."

I mentioned that a multiple vitamin each day would be a good idea for every inmate. They listened. I said that two a day would be even better; one at breakfast and one at lunch. They listened even more intently. They were either planning to break out with this information, or they really cared about their health.

It is somewhat surprising that the state does not give inmates a cheap daily nutritional supplement. It would save money in health-care expenses, thereby making the taxpayers happy to spend the three or four cents extra per person per day. But politicians and public don't want anything to do with an idea like that. "Why should convicted felons get free vitamins? I work hard to make an honest living and I have to buy them."

But weigh this fact: at least one in four inmates in New York State prisons tests positive for tuberculosis (TB). These are often multi-drug-resistant strains of TB at that. In some correctional facilities, the tuberculosis rate is nearly one in two. If you want to let prisoners infect each other and die, and if you consider that punishment to fit their many crimes, I will not contest it here. I remind you of this, however: even though you lock them up, nearly every inmate will get out eventually. Even without work-release or parole, you still cannot imprison everybody for life. And even if you could, you would still have the guards, nurses, cooks, and all other staff that work at the prison coming home each night to their families and their communities. This virtually guarantees the spread of viruses and bacteria outside of prison walls. Tuberculosis is well known to flourish when diet is poor, and there is also a connection with diet and most other contagious diseases. It is therefore economical for the taxpayer to keep inmates from getting sick.

I wrote a letter to the State about the TB problem in its prisons. The result was a written response from the central Department of Corrections office. It says that "we are doing everything possible to contain the spread of this virus." The letter is signed by a senior health official. Everyone knows that tuberculosis is not viral, it is bacterial. Well, almost everyone knows that.

Back to that big, scary inmate. He made eye contact with me more during my talk about wheat germ and vitamins than ever before. A number of classes later, everybody was filing out and the Big Guy lagged behind. He moved up close beside me.

"Can I talk to you for a minute?" he whispered. "I've been eating that stuff, that wheat germ, you told us about."

"How did you come up with it?"

"They sell it in the commissary," he answered. "They got those multivitamins too. Been taking them." There was an uncomfortable pause, and then he continued: "Well, I just wanted to tell you," he said, "that I've been taking those vitamins and eating that wheat germ for a couple of weeks now, and I feel more clear."

He put an unusual emphasis on the word *clear*, looking me straight in the eye. It finally dawned on me that this was a compliment, a thank you. "Oh, good!" I said. "Keep on doing it." From time to time, I have considered the benefits to society of having a man like that feeling more "clear." I think that reaching some form of clarity in prison might go a long way toward actually making them correctional institutions. Nutritional supplements could make it happen.

THE WONDERS OF PROPER NUTRITION

During my (RC) time as a jail doctor in Montana, I was the only doctor and the inmates had to adjust to my odd ways. Most inmates were in poor physical shape: there was a high percentage of alcoholism and most had terrible eating patterns, poor lifestyles, and glaring nutritional deficiencies. Strangely enough, I saw almost no infectious diseases other than mild viral respiratory illnesses.

One reason may be that every inmate got a multivitamin/mineral preparation and a minimum of 500 mg (one chewtab) of vitamin C each morning. I worked with the cook to get the healthiest diet we could while under the thumb of those who controlled the purse strings, who weren't interested in making changes. Most were in need of vitamin E, the B vitamins, or lots more vitamin C, depending on the medical complaint. I witnessed the "miracle" of vitamins C and E together as they quickly healed a tooth socket resulting from an extraction.

Many inmates had no idea what their medications were for, making nutrition education even more of a challenge. I also encouraged use of the exercise facilities. If I did gain their interest and they were in long enough, inmates often achieved good results. Many were able to get off of their medications, and I made sure they were not addicted to any narcotics or other habit-forming drugs before discharge. I was confident that at least some would take their newfound knowledge with them. This is a cycle that applies to everyone: start on the road to good health, start feeling better (both physically and mentally), and that reinforces your motivation to continue.

One inmate, who had made many visits to a Veterans Administration outpatient clinic when he was "outside" presented an interesting picture at his intake examination. He had a "furrowed tongue" and cracked lips that were almost magenta in color. He also had generalized dermatitis and complained of his bowels being chronically upset. After questioning him, I found that he had a lousy diet and imbibed alcohol liberally. These were two of the classic signs—the three "D's"—of pellagra, a disease caused by deficiency of niacin, with other B vitamins as cofactors: diarrhea and dermatitis. As I continued to converse with him, I began to see the third sign as well, a bit of dementia. His medical record showed visits to and prescriptions from each of the symptom-related clinics: gastrointestinal medication for the diarrhea (irritable bowel syndrome), psychiatric medication for his rather bizarre ideation, and drugs from a dermatology clinic. A short time on a B-complex supplement (100 mg of most of the B vitamins) and withdrawing his medications after a few days did wonders.

At a maximum-security prison in England, a team of Oxford scientists found that vitamin supplements reduced violent crime. Of 231 young adult prisoners studied, those taking nutritional supplements had an average 35 percent reduction in offenses. The authors concluded that "antisocial behavior in prisons, including violence, are reduced by vitamins, minerals, and essential fatty acids."[2]

Feeding Children Right to Keep Them Out of Trouble

Barbara Reed served as an Ohio probation officer for twenty years, where she developed a program on the relationship of diet and behavior. In 1982, she married biochemist Paul Stitt, who has conducted research for Tenneco Chemicals and the Quaker Oats Company and holds five U.S. patents. In 1997, the Stitts started a whole, fresh foods lunch program for the students of the Alternative High School in Appleton, Wisconsin. The results from improved nutrition: no dropouts, expulsions, drugs or weapons possessions, or suicides.

"As a probation officer, correcting the diet was my number one tool," says Barbara. In fact, improving nutrition worked so well that, after following up on people for a period of five years, she found that 89 percent had not gotten back into trouble.

Because of this success with diet and behavior when working with the courts, the Stitts decided to work with students and try to prevent problems. Providing fresh, whole foods to students improved their behavior and their learning ability, a winning combination. "We demonstrated the difference by requiring the teachers have a 'junk food day' every seven to eight weeks," says Barbara. "Within two hours, they had lost control of the class. Some students became hyper, others lethargic, others angry and violent in some cases. We required this to allow the children to understand that it was what they were putting in their mouth that was causing the problems in how they felt and behaved."[3]

According to the Stitts, the centerpiece of the meal should be whole-grain food, complemented with tasty vegetable dishes with fruit as an appetizer. Soup, salads, and breads make for very nutritionally complete meals. Meat is for flavoring. As Paul says, "Always do what you know is best for your body." They recommend feeding children fresh, whole fruits, vegetables, legumes, whole-grain breads and cereals, nuts, seeds, and water, and also lead them into good exercise, so they can be healthy and have a long, productive life. The artificially colored, sweetened cereals, soda, sweets, and products made with enriched white flour and sugar all cause children to be ill and unable to behave and learn.

SUMMARY

Like so many media stories, we accentuate the negative as we deal with the consequences of behavior. It is the "bad" that gets all the attention, because bad behavior spreads at home or in the classroom. It can be countered with "good" in a learned process. Good behavior patterns need to be established and bad patterns squelched sooner rather than later, before a child has reasoning power. The "tough love" concept is helpful. The bigger, wiser parent is the boss, who must be firm, fair, and confident in his or her approach to the child. No matter the age, when unacceptable behavior appears, evaluate the diet and basic vitamin needs and adjust in keeping with the advice in this book. Make certain that there are no obscure medical conditions that might be affecting behavior. Then, employ the biochemical boost provided by megadose vitamins, especially when the undesirable behavior comes in bursts.

PART FOUR

VITAMIN
THERAPY

CHAPTER 12

HIGH-DOSE VITAMIN C THERAPY

*"Vitamin C can truthfully be designated
as the antitoxic and antiviral vitamin."*
—CLAUS W. JUNGEBLUT, M.D.

"Vitamin deficiencies" are defined only as being manifest in deficiency diseases pinned down in the 1930s. Most conventional scientists and researchers don't accept the concept of "optimal" doses that promote health and prevent disease. They claim that those who advocate supplementation ignore the belief that a normal diet will provide adequate nutrients to avoid deficiencies. We don't ignore this statement—we reject it. What is "normal"? And if we can define *normal,* how do we achieve it? Five to seven pesticide-laden fruit and vegetable servings a day, plus processed foods devoid of many nutrients—are these part of a "normal" diet?

The no-supplement alternative of "eat a varied diet rich in fruits, vegetables, and whole grains" is very worthwhile if one is able to accomplish it. Try working all those vegetable and fruit servings into your daily cuisine. Polls show that fewer than 20 percent of Americans do this. Why? They can't find those foods or can't afford what they do find, so they are buying nutrient-free, cheap, processed junk food. This type of diet requires judicious supplementation just to meet basic nutritional requirements, particularly in growing children.

Our number one supplement for maintaining health and preventing disease in children is vitamin C. In the next chapter, we will discuss some additional vital supplements.

A HISTORY OF VITAMIN C RESEARCH

Decades of physicians' reports and controlled studies support the use of very large doses of ascorbate (vitamin C). Effective doses are high doses, often 1,000 times more than the standard U.S. Recommended Dietary Allowance (RDA) or Daily Reference Intake (DRI). It is a cornerstone of medical science that dose affects treatment outcome. This premise is accepted with pharmaceutical drug therapy, but apparently not with vitamin therapy, at least in conventional medical circles. Most conventional vitamin C research has used inadequate, low doses, which do not get clinical results.

Investigators using vitamin C in high doses have consistently reported excellent results. Many of these researchers were pioneers in the field of orthomolecular medicine. Unfortunately, the medical literature has ignored nearly seventy-five years of laboratory and clinical studies on high-dose ascorbate therapy. Dosage of tens of thousands of milligrams of vitamin C is the most unacknowledged successful research in medicine.

William J. McCormick, M.D. (1880–1968)

Over sixty years ago, Dr. McCormick saw vitamin C deficiency as the essential cause of, and effective cure for, numerous communicable illnesses. He was one of the very first to advocate injected, gram-sized doses of vitamin C as an antiviral and antibiotic.[1]

Dr. McCormick also noted that four out of five coronary cases in the hospital show vitamin C deficiency.[2] Vitamin C is essential to strengthen the walls of blood vessels, both small and large. A vitamin C–deficient artery can literally "bleed" into itself. If a blood clot forms, then a stroke may result. Over fifty years ago, Dr. McCormick found that the smoking of one cigarette "neutralizes in the body approximately 25 mg of ascorbic acid."[3] He recognized that cigarette smoking, in causing vitamin C deficiency, causes artery damage and cardiovascular disease. Thirty years later, Linus Pauling, Ph.D., and Matthias Rath would go on to demonstrate how vitamin C was a cure for cardiovascular disease.[4]

The U.S. National Institutes of Health is now interested in high doses of injected vitamin C as chemotherapy against cancer.[5] The medical journals and popular mass media report this as something new, somewhat promising, and definitely unproven. Yet, in 1954, Dr. McCormick noted that persons with cancer typically have exceptionally low levels of vitamin C in their tissues, a deficiency of approximately 4,500 mg.[6]

Frederick R. Klenner, M.D. (1907–1984)

For decades, Dr. Klenner treated patients with injections of vitamin C, ranging from 350 mg to 1,200 mg per kilogram of body weight per day. This amounts to very large doses of ascorbate: vitamin C at 350 mg/kg is about 20,000–35,000 mg per day for an adult; at 1,200 mg/kg, this is about 70,000–120,000 mg per day. Dr. Klenner successfully treated polio, pneumonia, and other serious infectious diseases.[7] He treated an astounding variety of diseases with massive doses of vitamin C: bladder infections, arthritis, leukemia, atherosclerosis, high cholesterol, diabetes, glaucoma, burns and secondary infections, heat stroke, heavy metal poisoning, chronic fatigue, and complications resulting from surgery. Additionally, he arrested and reversed multiple sclerosis with very high doses of vitamin C and other vitamins.[8]

Robert F. Cathcart, M.D. (1932–2007)

Since the 1960s, Dr. Cathcart successfully used large doses of vitamin C against pneumonia, hepatitis, and, more recently, AIDS.[9] He treated over 30,000 patients.

Hugh D. Riordan, M.D. (1932–2005)

Dr. Riordan successfully used large doses of intravenous vitamin C against cancer, beginning in the 1970s.[10] Dr. Riordan and colleagues have published on this for many years, but their work has been largely ignored.

VITAMIN C: IT'S ALL ABOUT DOSE

Our bodies cannot make vitamin C, although most animals can. We must get it from our food and from supplements. But how much do we really need? Persistent arguments on this question may be settled by looking at how much vitamin C animals manufacture in their bodies. The simple answer is quite a lot. Most animals make the human body-weight equivalent of 5,000–10,000 mg a day. It is unlikely that animals would have evolved to make this much vitamin C if they did not need it and use it. Indeed, cells in many human body tissues concentrate vitamin C by 25-fold or more over blood concentration.

Each person's need for vitamin C differs because of differences in genetics and individual biochemistry.[11] Further, our bodies undergo different stresses, and we certainly eat different foods. Therefore, the daily need for ascorbate to maintain health for an adult varies between 2,000–20,000 mg/day. Dr. Pauling personally took 18,000 mg of vitamin C daily. Although he was often ridiculed for this, it is interesting to note that Dr. Pauling had two more Nobel Prizes than any of his critics, and he died at age ninety-three.

When we are challenged with a viral infection, our need for vitamin C can rise dramatically, depending on the body's immune function, level of injury, infection, or environmental toxicity, such as cigarette smoke.[12] Ascorbate at sufficiently high doses can prevent viral disease and greatly speed recovery from an acute viral infection. Surprising to some, this was originally observed by physicians in the 1940s and has been verified and re-verified over the last half century by doctors who achieved quick and complete recovery in their patients with ascorbate megadoses.[13] The effective therapeutic dose is based on clinical observation and bowel tolerance. Clinical observation is essentially "taking enough C to be symptom free, whatever that amount may be." Bowel tolerance means exactly what you think it means: the amount that can be absorbed from the gut without causing loose stools.[14] Very high doses, in the range of 30,000–200,000 mg, divided up throughout the day, are remarkably nontoxic and have been documented by physicians as curing viral diseases including the common cold, flu, hepatitis, viral pneumonia, and even polio.[15]

Several mechanisms for vitamin C's antiviral effect are known or suggested from studies.[16] The antioxidant property of ascorbate promotes a reducing environment in the bloodstream and tissues, absorbing harmful free radical molecules and enhancing the body's response to oxidative stress from inflammation,[17] thereby helping to fight microbes and viruses that propagate in stressful conditions.[18] Ascorbate has been shown to have specific antiviral effects in which it inactivates the genetic RNA or DNA of viruses[19] or affects the assembly of the virus.[20]

Vitamin C is also involved in enhancing several functions of the immune system. Ascorbate can boost the production of interferon, an immune protein that helps prevent cells from being infected by a virus.[21] Ascorbate stimulates the activity of antibodies,[22] and in megadoses seems to have a role in mitochondrial energy production.[23] It can enhance phagocyte function, which is the body's mechanism for engulfing bacteria, removing viral particles and other unwanted debris.[24] White blood cells, involved in the body's defense against infections of all types, concentrate ascorbate up to eighty times plasma levels, which, if you take enough vitamin C, allows them to bring huge amounts of ascorbate to the site of the infection.[25] Many different components with important roles in the immune response—B cells, T cells, natural killer (NK) cells, and also cytokine production—are enhanced by ascorbate.[26] Additionally, vitamin C improves the immune response from vaccination.[27] And it reduces the incidence and severity of vaccination reactions if children have any sort of infection at the time of inoculation.[28]

Vitamin C at high doses is effective in preventing viral infection and enhancing recovery. When taken at an appropriate dose in a timely manner, ascorbate is our best tool for curing acute viral illness.

DIET IS NOT ENOUGH

It was more or less a normal lecture until I (AWS) started talking about vitamin C. I made routine mention that cooking destroys vitamin C. Presently, I added that almost all animals, such as rats, make their own vitamin C. Fully expecting to move on, I was stopped by a student question that I probably should have seen coming: "If rats make their own vitamin C, are rats a good source of vitamin C?"

"Yes," I answered, "If you eat your rats raw." Well, that's technically true, isn't it? The student then asked how much vitamin C is in a rat. You have to be ready for these things. "According to Lendon Smith, M.D., 'if we base our needs on the amounts other mammals manufacture . . . it comes to 2–4 grams daily in the unstressed condition. Under stress, 70 kg of rats make 15 grams of C.'"

So, we did some math. Though some are much larger, an average rat weighs about 0.25 kilograms, which works out to about 53 mg of vitamin C in a well-stressed 9-ounce rat. A glass of ready-to-drink orange juice provides 45 mg of vitamin C; the frozen concentrate provides more C (pasteurized, ready-to-serve orange juice typically contains 25 percent less vitamin C per serving than frozen concentrates). Of course, just because a rat makes 5 mg of vitamin C does not mean that all of it is in the rat at one time. A rat uses it. But then, orange juice loses it. In fact, the amount of vitamin C in ready-to-drink brands of orange juice can fall to zero within four weeks after opening.

Looks like you'd have to eat those rats raw after all. Although, let it be said that I do not recommend eating rats, be they raw, well-done, or otherwise.

Animals thrive on raw food, and they make their own vitamin C to boot. When they are eaten by carnivores, they *are* raw food. Raw foods (rats included) are a good source of vitamin C. Cooked foods aren't, because heat destroys vitamin C. Nutrition textbooks, plus McDonald's and all the other purveyors of french fries, can now stop claiming that fries provide vitamin C simply because potatoes do. By the time the fast-food potato is ultra-processed and dredged out of the deep fryer, the vitamin C is gone.

The moral of the story: we humans would do well to eat our food raw whenever practical. Not being much of a rat-eater myself, and having raised my children on a ratless diet, I'd recommend lots of salads and raw fruits and fresh, well-chewed nuts. Add to this whole grains and legumes (beans, peas, lentils), which you need to cook if you do not sprout them. Scrupulously clean raw milk, if you can get it, is excellent. If you can't, cheese and yogurt are very close to a raw food because of their high count of beneficial microorganisms.

Since we do cook so much of our food, and we are under stress and we do get sick, we truly need vitamin C supplementation. And though it is an excellent preventive, even a mostly raw diet does not provide enough ascorbate to cure serious illness. Therefore, take vitamin C with every meal, and between meals as well.

HOW TO USE VITAMIN C EFFECTIVELY

Remember the "fire triangle"? If you ever were a Boy Scout or went to a good wilderness camp, you know that to make a fire, you need three things: fuel, oxygen, and kindling temperature. With vitamin C therapy, the magic triangle is quantity, frequency, and duration. In this book, there has been ample discussion about "quantity." And "duration" is a no-brainer: take lots until you are well; and, of course, keep taking a maintenance dose. So, let's talk about that third, often overlooked, and very important leg of the triangle: frequency.

By dividing the dose all through the day, your absorption of ascorbate is greatly enhanced. You can achieve three times higher vitamin C blood concentrations with oral-dose vitamin C than has generally been believed. With an oral dose of 3 grams (3,000 mg) vitamin C every four hours, pharmacokinetics predicts peak plasma concentrations of 220 micromol/L.[29] This about four to six times typical vitamin C blood levels. Intravenous ascorbate is, of course, even better: concentrations of vitamin C from intravenous administration may be 140-fold higher than from maximum oral doses.

Take Enough C

There is a "trick" to treating illness with oral vitamin C: *take enough C to be symptom free, whatever the amount might be.* That is usually just under the amount that would result in loose bowels.

I (AWS) saw very high doses work time after time with children of all ages while I was a natural therapeutics consultant for thirty years and especially in the raising of my own kids. It is the only medication they had. When my daughter was four years old, she had a very bad cough. We endured it for two nights while doing what doctors typically suggest, strict bed rest and codeine cough syrup. Yet, she still was coughing after forty-eight hours. So, I started my daughter on a teaspoon (about 4,000 milligrams) of vitamin C crystals in juice every hour. When my wife returned home, the cough was gone. We continued to give her vitamin C for the rest of the day, and she remained quiet and comfortable. She had a total of 36,000 mg of C. During the night, the cough came back. We got up, gave her a teaspoon of vitamin C, and everyone was soon asleep once again. The next morning, the cough was back again, and we met it with vitamin C every hour. We kept that cough down by keeping her C up.

I tell you this to let you know that I've been there too. Those all-night battles for a sick child are really tough. Vitamin C is tough too, if you use enough. When you do, it really works, and everybody sleeps much better.

Here is another example of vitamin C in action: Ray, a primary care physician, brought his eleven-month-old son, Robbie, to me. The child had been very sick for over a week, and no one in their family had had any sleep in a long time. They were up night after night with this child, who had a high fever, glazed watery eyes, tons of thick watery mucus, and labored breathing. Robbie would not sleep and did little else but cry.

Robbie was under the care of a pediatrician who had been prescribing antibiotics, but the medication was clearly not working. This was all too apparent to Ray. "Twelve rounds of antibiotics for a baby under a year old, and all the doctor wants to do is give more antibiotics?" he said. "That makes no sense at all."

"Ray, antibiotics are a knee-jerk answer to a lot of things. There is a saying: 'When the only tool you have is a hammer, you tend to see every problem as a nail.'"

"Well, we've thoroughly tried the medical route and cooperated a hundred percent with the pediatrician, and Robbie is worse, not better," Ray said. "We have got to do something ourselves."

I promptly acquainted Ray with the vitamin C doctors mentioned earlier in this chapter.

"So, the bottom line is to give Robbie as much vitamin C as he can hold without having loose bowels," Ray said. And he did, too. It took 20,000 mg of vitamin C daily to cure a 20-pound baby of severe congestion, fever, and listlessness. That is 1,000 mg of vitamin C per pound per day (2,200 mg of C per kilogram body weight per day), nearly twice what Dr. Klenner customarily ordered for patients. Even at that huge amount, the baby never had diarrhea!

"Robbie was noticeably improved in under twelve hours, and slept through the first night." Ray told me two days later. "He was completely well in forty-eight hours."

Even without considering the harmful side effects of massive antibiotic therapy, we can see in this case the futility of repeated doses. Antibiotics are either going to work with the first or second round, or they are not going to work at all, period.

Taking enough C results in the three C's: patient comfort, low cost, and parental control. Without necessitating the use of invasive technology or the trauma of hospitalization, parents can regain confidence and mastery over illness to a degree that they might never have thought possible. But do not be overly surprised when vitamin C therapy is denounced as irresponsible. It takes some real ego strength for a parent to stand firm and say, "This is what I am going to do—I am going to use very high doses of vitamin C." The vitamin C doctors' shared knowledge of how it is done is the buttress that makes such a stance possible.

Calculating a High Dosage for Children

Vitamin RDAs for all ages are published on the Internet and to some extent are also found on vitamin bottles. In many cases, these widely quoted nutritional standards are, we think, much too low. They certainly are for therapeutic applications. Therefore, for high-dosage computations, the simplest approach is to use the child's weight as your principal guideline. In other words, ask yourself, "What percentage of an adult do we have here?" Figure a normal adult as 180

ACHIEVING A THERAPEUTIC LEVEL OF VITAMIN C

Frederick Klenner, M.D., used the following basic formula for estimating therapeutic vitamin C doses: 350 mg of vitamin C per kilogram of body weight per day (350 mg/kg/day).[30] A kilogram is 2.2 pounds.

BODY WEIGHT (POUNDS)	VITAMIN C (MG)	DOSES	AMOUNT PER DOSE (MG)
7–8	1,200	9	130–135
14–15	2,300	9	250
28	4,500	9	500
55	9,000	18	500
110	18,000	18	1,000
220	35,000	17–18	2,000

These quantities may seem high, but *Dr. Klenner actually used up to four times as much,* typically by injection. These are moderate oral doses. You may also give twice as many doses, with half as much vitamin C per dose.

Vitamin C may be given as a liquid, powder, tablet, or chewtab. Infants often prefer finely powdered, naturally sweetened chewable tablets, which may be crushed for easier ingestion. You may make your own liquid vitamin C daily by dissolving C powder in a small (1 ounce) dropper bottle and adding a sweetener, if necessary. Dr. Klenner recommended daily preventive doses, which might be about one-sixth of the above therapeutic amounts, divided into three daily doses. Injections of vitamin C may be arranged with your physician.

Persons with sensitivity to citrus fruits, tomatoes, or cranberries may feel more comfortable taking vitamin C as ascorbate, a non-acidic form of vitamin C. Calcium ascorbate is most frequently chosen (it is about 11 percent calcium); sodium ascorbate is most commonly used for intravenous administration or intramuscular injection. A transition down to a maintenance level (about 60 mg/kg/day) should be made gradually, over a period of a week or two.

pounds and divide from there. An eighteen-pound infant is one-tenth (10 percent) of an adult; a fifty-four-pound child is four-tenths (40 percent) of an adult. When in doubt, round up. This is because children are active and growing and generally need considerably more nutrition per pound body weight than adults do. As you read more about high-dose vitamin therapy, in this book and others like it, you can take the adult therapeutic level, use this fractional approach, and get a quick approximation to work with.

Help the Vitamins Go Down

Many readers may want to know, "Exactly how do you get that much vitamin C into a child?" As an alumnus of the "Mary Poppins School of Medicine," let me say that the answer is sugar. Yes, sugar, that universal bane of health writers. Sweet sugar is the way to get little kids to take lots of sour ascorbic acid. Of course, you can simply use children's chewable vitamin C. Many kinds are really delicious, but they are pricey. Pure ascorbic acid dissolved in sugar water is the cheapest solution there is.

Now, I am not suggesting that you gorge your offspring on sugar. I'm simply a realist: this is cheap, and it works. If you put vitamin C powder in really sweet natural fruit juice, that often does the trick too. Remember to put all the C in just some of the juice. A child is more apt to down a small amount because it looks easy. My older brother tried to teach me how to ride a bicycle by putting me on his. It did not work because I was afraid of being up too high. At a playground one day, I borrowed a little kid's tiny two-wheeler and taught myself to ride it in five minutes. Later, I could ride my brother's big bike just fine. So, put all the C in a small volume of sweetened liquid, and after it's gone down the hatch, immediately have on hand a "chaser" of sweet juice. Your children will correctly see this as the bribe it is. Reward their taste buds for bravely taking their C powder, and they will keep doing it. For especially tricky kids, offering a tasty dessert food (such as a bite of cake) for a chaser makes it a lot less likely to come back up at you. Just a spoonful of pastry helps the vitamins go down, and stay down.

THE PROBLEM OF ACIDITY

Vitamin C is commonly taken in large quantities to improve health and prevent asthma, allergies, viral infection, and heart disease. It is nontoxic and does not irritate the stomach as drugs like aspirin can. Yet, vitamin C is acidic, so what are the effects from taking large quantities? Ascorbic acid is a weak acid, only slightly stronger than vinegar. Can large quantities of a weak acid such as ascorbate cause problems in the body? The answer is, sometimes, in some situations. However, with some simple precautions, they can be avoided.

Acid in the Mouth

Any acid can etch the surfaces of your teeth. This is the reason the dentist cleans your teeth and warns about plaque, for acid generated by bacteria in the mouth can cause cavities. Cola soft drinks contain phosphoric acid, actually used by dentists to etch teeth before tooth sealants are applied. Like soft drinks, ascorbic acid will not cause etching of teeth if only briefly present. Often, vitamin C tablets are coated with a tableting ingredient such as magnesium stearate, which prevents the ascorbate from dissolving immediately. Swallowing a vitamin C tablet without chewing it prevents its acid from harming tooth enamel.

Chewable vitamin C tablets are popular because they taste sweet and so are good for encouraging children to take their vitamin C. However, some chewable vitamin C tablets can contain sugar and ascorbic acid that, when chewed, is likely to stick in the crevices of your teeth. So, after chewing a vitamin C tablet, rinse with water or brush your teeth. Also, you can select non-acidic vitamin C chewables, readily available in stores.

Stomach Acidity

People with sensitive stomachs may report discomfort when large doses of vitamin C are taken at higher levels (1,000–3,000 mg or more every twenty minutes). In this case, the ascorbic acid in the stomach can build up enough acidity to cause heartburn or a similar reaction. On the other hand, many people report no problems with acidity even when taking 20,000 mg in an hour. The acid normally present in the stomach, hydrochloric acid (HCl), is dozens of times more acidic than vitamin C. When one has swallowed a huge amount of ascorbate, the digestive tract is taking it up into the bloodstream as fast as it can, but it may still take a while to do so. Some people report that they seem to sense ascorbic acid tablets "sitting" at the bottom of the stomach as they take time to dissolve. It is fairly easy to fix the problem by using buffered ascorbate or taking ascorbic acid with food or liquids in a meal or snack. When the amount of vitamin C ingested is more than the gut can absorb, the ascorbate attracts water into the intestines, creating a laxative effect. This saturation intake is called "bowel tolerance." One should reduce the amount (by 20–50 percent) when this occurs.

Acid Balance in the Body

Does taking large quantities of an acid, even a weak acid like ascorbate, tip the body's acid balance (pH) and cause health problems? No, because the body actively and constantly controls the pH of the bloodstream. The kidneys regulate the acid in the body over a long time period, hours to days, by selectively excreting either acid or basic components in urine. Over a shorter time period, minutes to hours, if the blood is too acidic, the autonomic nervous system increases the rate of breathing, thereby removing more carbon dioxide from the blood, reducing its acidity. Some foods can indirectly cause acidity. For example, when more protein is eaten than necessary for maintenance and growth, it is metabolized into acid, which must be removed by the kidneys, generally as uric acid. In this case, calcium and/or magnesium are excreted along with the acid in the urine, which can deplete the body's supplies. However, because ascorbic acid is a weak acid, we can tolerate a lot before it will much affect the body's acidity. Although there have been allegations about vitamin C supposedly causing kidney stones, there is no evidence for this, and its acidity and diuretic tendency actually tends to reduce kidney stones in most people who are prone to them.

Forms of Vitamin C

Ascorbate comes in many forms, each with a particular advantage. Ascorbic acid is the least expensive and can be purchased as tablets, timed-release tablets, or powder. The larger tablets (1,000–1,500 mg) are convenient and relatively inexpensive. Timed-release tablets contain a long-chain carbohydrate that delays the stomach in dissolving the ascorbate, which is then released over a period of hours. This may have an advantage for maintaining a high level in the bloodstream. Ascorbic acid powder or crystals can be purchased in bulk relatively inexpensively. Pure powder is more quickly dissolved than tablets and therefore can be absorbed somewhat faster by the body.

Buffered Ascorbate—A fraction of a teaspoon of sodium bicarbonate (baking soda) has long been used as a safe and effective antacid that immediately lowers stomach acidity. When sodium bicarbonate is added to ascorbic acid, the bicarbonate fizzes (emitting carbon dioxide), which then releases the sodium to neutralize the acidity of the ascorbate.

Calcium ascorbate can be purchased as a powder and readily dissolves in water or juice. In this buffered form, ascorbate is completely safe for the mouth and sensitive stomach and can be applied directly to the gums to help heal infections. It is a little more expensive than the equivalent ascorbic acid and bicarbonate but more convenient. Calcium ascorbate has the advantage of being non-acidic. It has a slightly metallic taste and is astringent but not sour like ascorbic acid. A 1,000 mg dose of calcium ascorbate contains about 110 mg of calcium. Other forms of buffered ascorbate include sodium ascorbate and magnesium ascorbate. Most adults need 800–1,200 mg of calcium and 400–600 mg of magnesium daily. The label on the bottle of all these buffered ascorbates details how much "elemental" mineral is contained in a teaspoonful. They cost a little more than ascorbic acid.

Buffered forms of ascorbate are often better tolerated at higher doses than ascorbic acid, but they appear not to be as effective for preventing the acute symptoms of a cold. This may be because, after they are absorbed, they must absorb an electron from the body to become effective as native ascorbate.

Liposomal Vitamin C—Recently, a revolutionary form of ascorbate has become available: vitamin C packaged inside nano-scale phospholipid spheres ("liposomes"), much like a cell membrane protects its contents. The lipid spheres protect the vitamin C from degradation by the environment and are absorbed more quickly into the bloodstream. Liposomes are also known to facilitate intracellular uptake of their contents, which can cause an added clinical impact when delivering something such as vitamin C. This form is supposed to be up to tenfold more absorbable than straight ascorbic acid. It is more expensive than ascorbic acid tablets or powder.

Ascorbyl Palmitate—Ascorbyl palmitate is composed of an ascorbate molecule bound to a palmitic acid molecule. It can dissolve in either water or fat (amphipathic), such as the fatty acids in cell membranes. It is widely used as an antioxidant in processed foods and in topical creams, where it is thought to be more stable than vitamin C. However, when ingested, the ascorbate component of ascorbyl palmitate appears to decompose into the ascorbate and palmitic acid molecules, so its special amphipathic quality is lost. It is also more expensive than ascorbic acid.

Natural Ascorbate—Natural forms of ascorbate derived from plants are also available. Acerola, the "Barbados cherry," contains a large amount of vitamin C (depending on its ripeness) and was traditionally used to fight off colds. Tablets of vitamin C purified from acerola or rose hips are generally low dose and considerably more expensive than ascorbic acid. Although some people strongly advocate this type, many have claimed that these forms are no better than pure commercial ascorbate. Bioflavonoids, antioxidants found in citrus fruits or rose hips, are often added to vitamin C supplements and are thought to improve uptake and utilization. However, tablets often do not contain enough bioflavonoids to make much difference.

NEUTRALIZING ACIDITY

To comfort all sensitive children's stomachs, buffer any excess acidity with a combination of calcium, food, and liquid. You can also buy non-acidic vitamin C, which is especially tooth-friendly and an important consideration in purchasing chewable tablets. But whether they're ingesting chewables or powder, non-acidic or not, get your children into the habit of rinsing their mouths with water after each dose.

You can neutralize vitamin C's acidity by adding a little baking soda (sodium bicarbonate) to the juice or water that you give with it. There is an additional payoff with this technique: harmless (but fun) carbon dioxide. As a boy, I liked to make baking-soda CO_2 fire extinguishers almost as much as I liked making the fires to extinguish. All you do is float a little container of baking soda in a big bottle of a weak acid. (We commandeered Mom's kitchen vinegar jug when she wasn't looking, which was seldom.) Attach a small hose and turn the bottle over—foam everywhere!

So, when you add baking soda to a solution of vitamin C powder (also a weak acid), you might want to stir it up to release the carbon dioxide. What is really fun is to give your kids a bicarbonate of soda rinse right after they drink C powder in juice. They'll get a mouthful of fizz. (Or mix the two together and deliberately create a bubbly drink!)

Why the comparison with vinegar? Because vinegar, considered a weak acid, is actually more acidic than ascorbic acid. Vinegar has an acidity of between 2.5 and 3.5 on the pH scale. (The lower the pH number, the greater the acidity.) The stomach contains a much stronger acid and therefore has a very low pH, usually between 1 and 2. The most concentrated ascorbic acid solution you could make might have a pH of about 3.5 to 4 (100 to 1,000 times weaker than acidity of the normal human stomach).

ABOUT "OBJECTIONS" TO VITAMIN C THERAPY

In massive doses, vitamin C stops a cold within hours, stops influenza in a day or two, and stops viral pneumonia (pain, fever, cough) in two or three days. It is a highly effective antihistamine, antiviral, and antitoxin. It reduces inflammation and lowers fever. Administered intravenously, ascorbate kills cancer cells without harming healthy tissue. Therefore, many people wonder, in the face of statements like these, why the medical profession has not embraced vitamin C therapy with open arms. Probably the main roadblock to widespread examination and utilization of this all-too-simple technology is the equally widespread belief that there *must* be unknown dangers to tens of thousands of milligrams of ascorbic acid. Yet, since the time megascorbate therapy was introduced in the late 1940s by Dr. Klenner, there has been an especially safe and extremely effective track record to follow. Still, for some, questions remain.

Is 2,000 mg per day of vitamin C a megadose?

No. Decades ago, Linus Pauling and Irwin Stone showed that most animals make at least that much (or more) per equivalent human body weight per day.[31] Then, why has the government set the "Safe Upper Limit" for vitamin C at 2,000 mg per day? Perhaps the reason is ignorance. According to nationwide data compiled by the American Association of Poison Control Centers, vitamin C (and the use of any other dietary supplement) does not kill anyone.[32]

Does vitamin C damage DNA?

No. If vitamin C harmed DNA, why do most animals make (not eat, but *make*) 2,000–10,000 mg of vitamin C per equivalent human body weight per day? Evolution would never so favor anything that harms vital genetic material. White blood cells and male reproductive fluids contain unusually high quantities of ascorbate. Living, reproducing systems love vitamin C.

Does vitamin C cause low blood sugar, vitamin B_{12} deficiency, birth defects, or infertility?

Vitamin C does not cause birth defects, infertility, or miscarriage. "Harmful effects have been mistakenly attributed to vitamin C, including hypoglycemia, rebound scurvy, infertility, mutagenesis, and destruction of vitamin B_{12}. Health professionals should recognize that vitamin C does not produce these effects."[33]

Does vitamin C cause kidney stones?

No. The myth of the vitamin C–caused kidney stones is rivaled in popularity only by the Loch Ness Monster. A factoid-crazy medical media often overlooks the fact that Dr. McCormick demonstrated that vitamin C actually prevents the formation of kidney stones. He did so in 1946, when he published a paper on the subject.[34] His work was confirmed by University of Alabama professor of medicine Emanuel Cheraskin, M.D. Dr. Cheraskin showed that vitamin C inhibits the formation of oxalate stones.[35]

A recent large-scale, prospective study followed 85,557 women for fourteen years and found no evidence that vitamin C causes kidney stones.[36] Other research reports that "even though a certain part of oxalate in the urine derives from metabolized ascorbic acid, the intake of high doses of vitamin C does not increase the risk of calcium oxalate kidney stones. . . . (I)n the large-scale Harvard Prospective Health Professional Follow-Up Study, those groups in the highest quintile of vitamin C intake (greater than 1,500 mg per day) had a lower risk of kidney stones."[37]

"I started using vitamin C in massive doses in patients in 1969," stated Dr. Cathcart. "By the time I read that ascorbate should cause kidney stones, I had clinical evidence that it did not cause kidney stones, so I continued prescribing massive doses to patients. Up to 2006, I estimate that I have put 25,000 patients on massive doses of vitamin C and none have developed kidney stones."

Does vitamin C narrow arteries or cause atherosclerosis?

Abram Hoffer, M.D., has said: "I have used vitamin C in megadoses with my patients since 1952 and have not seen any cases of heart disease develop even after decades of use. . . . The fact is that vitamin C *decreases* plaque formation according to many clinical studies. Some critics ignore the knowledge that thickened arterial walls in the absence of plaque formation indicate that the walls are becoming stronger and therefore less apt to rupture."[38] Researchers investigated how smooth muscle cells go from the media (middle of artery tissue) into the intima (inside surface) and grow, narrowing the lumen

(open space) and showed that vitamin C prevents this and is a valuable tool to reduce such growth.[39]

So why the flurry of anti–vitamin C reporting in the mass media?
Negative news sells newspapers and magazines and pulls in television
viewers. Positive *drug* studies do get headlines, of course, but positive vitamin studies do not. While this is not likely due to any grand
conspiracy, it is nevertheless an enormous public health problem.
The fact is that 150 million Americans take supplemental vitamin C
every day. This is as much a political issue as a scientific issue. What
would happen if everybody took vitamins? Perhaps doctors, hospital
administrators, and pharmaceutical salespeople would all be lining
up for their unemployment checks.

SUMMARY

The "dumb animal" is, biochemically speaking, pretty smart: it automatically produces the amount of vitamin C needed to correct the
results of stress that it is enduring. It doesn't have to think about it.
We primates, along with the guinea pig and the fruit bat, are unique
in that we have lost our ability to make vitamin C on demand from
the simplest of substrates, glucose. Medicines are given as a specific
amount, based on weight of the patient, for a specific target. Vitamin
C is not a medicine, but it can do what no medicine can.

We should be on a regular, divided, daily dose amount that promotes optimal health, while being prepared to provide megadoses
when under added stress or illness. Try to recognize the stressors you
and your child face in everyday life—physical exhaustion, thwarting
or undergoing infection, allergy reactions, and mental and emotional stress. And take enough vitamin C to be symptom free, whatever
the amount may be.

CHAPTER 13

VITAMIN D AND
OTHER SUPPLEMENTS

"One grandmother is worth two M.D.s"
—ROBERT MENDELSOHN, M.D.

he U.S. Recommended Dietary Allowance (RDA)/Dietary Reference Intakes (DRIs) are too low and most should be raised immediately, says an independent panel of physicians, academics, and
researchers. The Independent Vitamin Safety Review Panel writes,
"Government-sponsored nutrient recommendations, such as the US
RDA/DRIs, are not keeping pace with recent progress in nutrition
research. While current official recommendations for vitamin A, iron,
calcium, and some other nutrients are generally adequate, the public
has been asked to consume far too little of many other key nutrients.
Inadequate intake, and inadequate standards by which to judge
intake, have resulted in widespread nutrient inadequacy, chronic disease, and an undernourished but overweight population."[1] Citing a
large number of physician reports and clinical studies, the IVSRP
called for substantial increases in daily intake of the B-complex
vitamins; vitamins C, D, and E; and the minerals selenium, zinc, magnesium, and chromium. "Raising the RDA/DRI will save lives and
improve health," the panel said. "Clinical and subclinical nutrient
deficiencies are among the main causes of our society's greatest
health-care problems. Cancer, cardiovascular disease, mental illness,
and other diseases are caused or aggravated by poor nutrient intake.
The good news is that scientific evidence shows that adequately high

consumption of nutrients helps prevent these diseases." The panel concluded by stating: "In the past, over-conservative government-sponsored standards have encouraged dietary complacency. People have been led to believe that they can get all the nutrients they need from a 'balanced diet' of processed foods. That is not true. For ade-

OPTIMUM VITAMIN INTAKE RECOMMENDATIONS FOR ADULTS, TEENS AND CHILDREN

	ADULT (180 LBS)	TEEN (90 LBS)	CHILD (45 LBS)
Vitamin A	5,000 IU (as retinol, the oil form) Plus: 20,000 IU (as carotene)	5,000 IU (as retinol) Plus: 10,000 IU (as carotene)	5,000 IU (as retinol) Plus: 5,000 IU (as carotene)
Vitamin B-Complex			
Thiamine (B$_1$)	75 mg	50 mg	25 mg
Riboflavin (B$_2$)	75 mg	50 mg	25 mg
Niacinamide (B$_3$)	250 mg	200 mg	150 mg
Pyridoxine (B$_6$)	75 mg	50 mg	25 mg
Cobalamin (B$_{12}$)	125 mcg	125 mcg	75 mcg
Biotin	0.7 mg	0.7 mg	0.3 mg
Pantothenic Acid	150 mg	100 mg	50 mg
Folate	800 mcg	400 mcg	200 mcg
Vitamin C	6,000 mg	4,000 mg	2,000 mg
Vitamin D	3,000 IU	3,000 IU	1,000 IU
Vitamin E	600 IU	400 IU	200 IU

Some hints:

Vitamin A: There is no limit on carotene. Obtain lots of it from orange and green vegetables and their juices.

B-complex: The easiest way is to use a comprehensive B-complex supplement. Teens: One high-potency balanced B-complex supplement per day. Children: One lower potency, or half a high-potency, tablet daily.

Vitamin C: Easy rule of thumb: the child's age in grams, divided by four. (Examples: Sixteen-year-old: 4 g (4,000 mg) per day; Six-year old: 1.5 g (1,500 mg) per day. Give in at least three divided doses.

quate vitamin and mineral intake, a diet of unprocessed, whole foods, along with the intelligent use of nutritional supplements, is more than just a good idea: it is essential."

Based on this and other modern assessments, we recommend that parents give their children more than the RDA of vitamins. That is why we suggest multivitamins/minerals, plus extra vitamins C, D, and E.

MULTIVITAMIN/MULTIMINERAL

We have emphasized vitamin C in this book for the same reason Nobel Prize–winner Linus Pauling did: it is especially important, safe, and effective. Vitamin C is, of all the nutrients, the one most likely to be lacking in a typical child's diet. It is also the one that is needed in the highest quantity for optimum preventive health and for rapid healing during illness.

However, no major league pitcher ever won a World Series alone. It takes a village of vitamin variety to raise a child. All nutrients are important, but most kids' diets provide ample protein, carbohydrates, and fats. Minerals and vitamins are sparse in processed foods. We therefore recommend that every child take a good multivitamin/multimineral preparation every day, preferably twice a day. As the distinguished vitamin researcher Dr. Roger J. Williams said over a half-century ago, it is best to have nutritional insurance. It is also economical, as a combination preparation gives you the most for the least money in the fewest tablets. Two multiples each day will provide a fairly good quantity of the B-complex vitamins and vitamin A. It will not provide enough vitamin D or E; these should be taken in addition, every day. Go for the full assortment, since nutrients work in concert.

VITAMIN D

"Turn off that TV and get outside!" Those dread words of my (AWS) mother's were the bane of my idea of an ideal childhood: plant oneself in front of the television and stay there. Not in my parents' house. Weekday afternoon or Saturday morning cartoons were out and playing outside was in. When we pleaded that none of our friends were outside, my mom said, "They'll see you and they'll come out." That's true; eventually they did, after they were done watching TV. When I got home from summer camp, one of my dad's highest compliments was, "It's about time you got some color on you." Every photo I've ever seen of myself as a kid shows that I was a platinum-haired, sun-bleached blondie, with a nice tan. Things are different today; we hear every mother (and practically all doctors) say, "Put on your sunscreen!"

The pendulum has swung too far. Total avoidance of sunlight is a bad idea. Sunlight is not merely good for our bones, but it is also very good for the rest of us. Sunlight and the vitamin D it gives us relieves depression; reduces risk of type 1 diabetes, rheumatoid arthritis, and multiple sclerosis; lowers blood pressure; and prevents cancer of the prostate, breast, ovaries, and digestive tract.

The kids of my generation baked all day in the sun, in the back yard or at the ballpark or beach. We covered up, if at all, only enough to keep the sun out of our eyes while catching a fly ball or perhaps to prevent burning. Sun block? Never heard of it. As a result, we probably got more sun than is safe. Moderates catch it from both ends. Sun-worshippers and tanning-booth shareholders think we need more sun, while even ten minutes of unprotected exposure to full sun three times a week is too much for the American Academy of Dermatology.[2]

Attention paid to vitamin D has been cyclical, in step with prevailing attitudes concerning nutrition and medicine. Even in the past decades of abysmal lack of nutrition knowledge, we could find those who understood the relationship of vitamin D to the classic deficiency disease, rickets. In my training, eons ago, medical students were made aware of the signs of rickets in infants—bow legs and an abnormally shaped rib cage, among others. Parents also got the message and gave their children (whether they liked it or not) cod liver oil, rich in vitamins A and D. As children, we learned why we had to take the awful stuff and that is wasn't too bad if mixed with something pleasant tasting. I think infants were spared from suffering this disease because mothers were being instructed to provide sun exposure for their infants. This attitude about the health benefits of sun was reflected in the establishment of sanatoriums (sun therapy) for the treatment of chronic diseases, especially tuberculosis.

The knowledge I (RC) have gained about vitamin D is from an attitude that (1) I know this is good stuff, and (2) I want to learn all I can about it and pass it on to all who will listen. Medicine, until recently, has tried every trick to discredit vitamins, including D. Now, after so very many years of neglect, the media bombards us with messages of vitamin D deficiency and its detrimental effect on the immune system, and I am amazed at how ignorant all age groups are about rickets. It is time to reinvent the wheel. On the other hand, there are studies presented, constantly, of the immune system boost from vitamin D.

As early as 1918, experimental vitamin D deficiency in dogs was created to produce rickets. By 1931, vitamin D was isolated. But cod (or other fish) liver oil remained the food source of choice. In the 1940s, a precursor to the active form of vitamin D, D_3, was added to milk (400 IU per quart). Prior to that, D_2 was developed as a food supplement to fortify other foods, so there was no more need to gag on cod liver oil. By the mid-1950s, a water-soluble form of vitamin D was universally prescribed for infants, in keeping with the pediatric literature, which was replete with nutrition articles. Inexplicably, a shift away from nutrition education began. What had worked for generations so effectively was abandoned. Maybe it was all those new drug advertisements that had something to do with it.

Forms of Vitamin D

The way vitamin D is made, stored, and utilized in our bodies is unique. That dreaded but marvelous substance, cholesterol, forms the base of a derivative that resides in the fat cells just under the skin. When skin is exposed to ultraviolet (UV) rays from the sun, this derivative is transformed to D_3. Diet-derived D_2 and D_3 each undergo changes in the liver and the kidneys to form both a non-active storage form of the vitamin and the active form (1,25-dihydroxy-vitamin D). In many tissues of our bodies, there are receptors for both forms.

The active form of vitamin D is a steroid, which puts it in a class with other steroids, such as hormones. Since we can get our vitamin D from sources other than diet, some say it is not a vitamin. But if the sun doesn't shine or we avoid sun exposure by clothing, occupation, or sunblock lotions, we must have a dietary source. In latitudes north of San Francisco or south of Buenos Aires, Argentina, UV radiation is very feeble for at least six months of the year. Natural food sources, except for the fish liver oils, are relatively meager.

We are left with the commercial D_3 and D_2 forms that don't seem all that attractive when we learn how they are made. Animal skins

THE OFFICIAL RECOMMENDED DIETARY ALLOWANCE (RDA) FOR VITAMIN D IS TOO LOW

(Adapted from material written by William B. Grant, Ph.D.)

Due to current lifestyles in the United States, most people do not spend sufficient time in the sun to produce the higher serum vitamin D levels associated with optimal health. African Americans are particularly vulnerable to low levels due to their darker skin, which reduces the amount of ultraviolet B (UVB) radiation that reaches the lower epidermis to produce previtamin D. African-Americans have a 25 percent higher mortality rate than Caucasians, and this difference may be explained in terms of lower serum D levels. Solar UVB is an excellent source of vitamin D during about half the year. The way to take advantage of the sun as a source of vitamin D is to expose as much of the body as possible without sunscreen near solar noon (the time when one's shadow is shorter than one's height) for 10–30 minutes, depending on skin pigmentation, being careful not to turn pink or red or to burn.[3]

Supplements represent an efficient way to obtain sufficient vitamin D. African-Americans should consider taking 3,000 international units (IU) per day while Caucasians should consider taking 2,000

are treated with organic solvents that extract the cholesterol derivative (7-dehydrocholesterol, the same precursor that resides under our
skin), which is then exposed to UV radiation to form D_3. D_2, said to
be derived from plant or "food" sources, occurs naturally in some
yeasts and fish, but most of it is obtained from UV radiation of cholesterol derivatives in foods like milk. Cholesterol extracted from the
lanolin of sheep wool, after going through many chemical processes
and UV radiation, can generate D_2. D_3 has greater activity than D_2,
but both are still in use. The large-dose vitamin D in use now, as a
readily available supplement, is the D_3 form.

IU per day. The current dietary guideline, approximately 600 IU per
day, is a slight and recent increase over the amount of vitamin D in
a spoonful of cod liver oil, which prevented rickets.

There are few adverse effects of vitamin D. With whole-body
exposure to the sun, one can make at least 10,000 IU per day in a
short time. Adverse effects such as hypercalcemia have been found
in general only for 20,000–40,000 IU per day for very long periods.
However, those with certain diseases (adenoma of the parathyroid
gland, granulomatous diseases, lymphoma, sarcoidosis, and tuberculosis) should limit their vitamin D intake, because the body's
innate immune system produces too much 1,25-dihydroxyvitamin D
in the serum, which can raise serum calcium levels too high.

Several studies have examined how much mortality rates and
economic burdens of disease could be lowered if the population had
more vitamin D. These studies were for Western Europe, Canada,
the Netherlands, and the United States. They generally found that
mortality rates could be reduced by about 15 percent. During
pregnancy and lactation, women should be taking about 6,000 IU
per day.

*William B. Grant earned his doctorate in physics at the University of Cal-
ifornia, Berkeley. He is the director of the Sunlight, Nutrition and Health
Research Center, in San Francisco, and has authored or co-authored over
180 papers in peer-reviewed journals.*

Uses of Vitamin D

The most well known use of the active form of vitamin D, 1,25 D, is its role in bone metabolism. Our bones are a reservoir for calcium, which has many more essential functions than just bone metabolism. If calcium intake is inadequate, or if absorption is poor, the calcium blood level will fall. If the fall is too severe, terrible consequences ensue (tetany, death). Help comes in the form of a hormone released from the parathyroid glands that activates 1,25 D. This reaction quickly relieves the low blood calcium problem, but the calcium is taken from the bone reservoir. The parathyroid hormone also allows enhanced absorption of calcium from the gut, in conjunction with vitamin D. While it causes bone breakdown, it also stimulates the production of bone cells (osteoblasts) to provide new bone growth. This entire metabolic loop is designed as a stop-gap measure and cannot be kept in place for the long term, because the parathyroid glands will continually put out too much hormone and bones will deteriorate. The loop makes it hard to achieve toxic levels, since reserve components of the vitamin are activated only as needed.

Fortunately, long before the mechanism of vitamin D metabolism was understood, doctors and nutrition scientists gave sound prevention-oriented advice. Consequently, we didn't see rickets. It seems that a long period of complacency followed, without reminders of the grave consequences of vitamin D deficiency. Neither did we have an understanding of vitamin D receptors in the many tissues other than bone. Vitamin D, attached to these receptors, regulates genes responsible for the health of the target organ. Some infants with rickets have heart failure that can be successfully treated and should have been prevented with vitamin D. Besides heart muscle, deficiency affects skeletal muscle and the immune system. Antioxidant production involved in quelling free radical production seems to parallel vitamin D production from the skin. For the last few years it seems a new use for this "cure-all" vitamin turns up every week. Are these findings new or have they just been ignored for decades?

Vitamin D and the Sun

We have partially described the cyclical attitude concerning sun expo-sure. A big change was brought about by the advent of UV-blocking sunscreen lotions used to prevent skin cancer. The feared skin cancers have a relationship to sun exposure. Some develop from precancer-ous lesions, such as actinic keratoses, which result from exposure to the shorter "burn" UVB rays (as compared to the longer UVA rays). The vague part of this relationship has to do with when the exposure occurred, the intensity, and which UV rays cause what types of can-cer. Most sunscreens used over the past decades blocked only the sun-burn-producing UVB rays. Another question is: How can malignant melanoma, which may rarely occur in such covered up areas as between the toes or on the labia, be related to sun exposure? Potent sun exposure may have taken place decades before these skin cancers appear. Gradually acquiring a tan, without burning, produces a very effective sunscreen yet allows the production of vitamin D, which can act as a boost for the immune system and cancer prevention.

We have not had sufficient time, or enough honest evaluation, to evaluate the use of sunscreen. There is no question that sunburn damages the skin's connective tissue as bad as tobacco exposure, pro-ducing deep wrinkles. I think, in general, cautious sun exposure trumps indiscriminate use of sunscreen. But it is much harder for very fair-skinned people to acquire that gradual, protective tan. Facial protection may well be needed during sunny months or when the sun's rays are reflected off of snow or water. From personal observation, I see a reduction in the formation of the lesions that lead to skin cancers, due to following the current high-dose vitamin D recommendations. In time, this should lead to reducing the inci-dence of skin cancer.

Taking Vitamin D

One advantage of vitamin D supplementation is that it sidesteps the whole sunblock versus sun worship argument. The amount of recom-mended vitamin D has cycled between extremes. Giving 400 IU of vitamin D to infants to prevent rickets was a universal recommendation in the 1950s. This, coupled with fortified infant formulas, worked pretty well. However, breastfed infants could suffer from deficiency of vitamin D. It seems that breast milk vitamin D levels plateau at a low level, no matter what the mother's intake may be. Strangely, recommendations for children and adults have been even as low as 200 IU daily. Complacency due to food supplementation was highlighted in 2009, by a spokesperson for the American Academy of Pediatrics, who stated that they thought that it was strange that physicians were seeing a return of rickets, even though vitamin D fortification of milk had been in place for many years. Apparently, the connection hadn't been made that many children preferred soda to milk or that only a low percentage of infants were being prescribed,

A GOOD USE OF VITAMIN B$_{12}$

In the mid-1960s, I (RC) attended a pediatric education meeting in Los Angeles. One of the speakers was a pediatrician from Beverly Hills and I admit to misjudging him, at first, as a "ritzy" doctor to the stars. Was I wrong! This man searched the foreign literature for useful pediatric "pearls" and told his audience of one he had found in the German literature.

He presented cases of what he called non-icteric (no jaundice) hepatitis, which was not due to the usual viruses of "hepatitis" but was related to virus infections such as influenza B strains or coxsackie virus (or the liver's reaction to them). The key diagnostic sign is a tender liver. Patients seek care because of problems associated with hepatitis: nausea, poor appetite, epigastric stomachache, a feeling of intense fatigue and weakness, with accompanying depression. The cure was provided by an intramuscular injection of 1,000 mcg (1 cc) of B$_{12}$ and the result was dramatic. Many times, the doctor had noted that when his pediatric patient was diagnosed, the patient's mother was also found to have a tender liver and to have suffered the same symptoms, perhaps several weeks previously.

or otherwise taking, a vitamin D supplement. Sun exposure was not even considered to be a factor.

In this explosive upswing in support of vitamin D, we are witnessing a complete turnabout in the attitude of the medical establishment. For decades, while published medical studies attempted to discredit the use of vitamin C or vitamin E, occasionally an article would appear that warned physicians of the danger of vitamin D toxicity. Such a study ignored the fact that "toxicity" was based on administering many thousands of international units (IU) over weeks of time but then concluding from this that anything over 800 IU for an adult (less for infants) was to be considered toxic. As late as 1998, we hit all-time lows of vitamin D recommendations: 200 IU for infants and children and adults up to age fifty-one; for those older than fifty-one,

I used this newfound knowledge and discovered that this syndrome frequently occurred during winter influenza B epidemics and summer coxsackie ("summer sore throat") epidemics. Since I was a victim of the influenza B–associated variety, I became a firm believer. One feisty ten-year-old patient, who came from a broken family, had been accompanied by his dad when I diagnosed the problem and he took the appropriate treatment without a whimper. I told him he should start to feel better in just a couple of days, but if he still felt bad after a week, he might need another shot. About a week later, he came into my office on his own after school, saying he felt better but wanted another shot. This from the same spunky kid who, at a tender age, described his problem with sugar ingestion as making him feel "spacey," a very apt term.

Some of the new doctors on the staff of our local hospital are more knowledgeable about nutritional medicine than the "old guard" medicos. I want parents to know that they should not feel anxious about engaging their doctors in discussion of vitamin therapy versus standard therapy. If the doctor isn't willing to listen, he or she should be replaced with one who will.

400–600 IU. Fortunately, by 2009, the infant recommendation returned to 400 IU per day. But there still is not a complete consensus concerning the toxic level.

A complete change of attitude is illustrated by a New Zealand study in which megadoses of vitamin D_3 were given to elderly patients in three different ways: a loading dose of 500,000 IU, a loading dose plus 50,000 IU per month, or just the 50,000 IU per month. Levels were highest from the second regimen, but even the third one was adequate, just slower in achieving high levels. The conclusion was that all regimens were safe.[4] In the northern United States, physicians are giving vitamin D–deficient elderly folks in rest homes 50,000 IU three times a week for several weeks, just to catch up and relieve deficiency. Having toxicity fears ever most in mind for so many years, I am waiting for the first condemning breakthrough news flash. Frankly, I don't think I will ever see it.

Vitamin D is good for you and your child. We recommend 1,000 IU per day for a child old enough to be able to swallow a little pill through pre-adolescence, and then even more for teens. For adults, the optimum level may be 4,000 IU per day or even more. As this is being written, the dose ceiling rises in exponential fashion, so keep tuned. Even the "experts" can't keep ahead of the recommendations. Capsule, tablet, or liquid is fine.

VITAMIN E

We used to prick both ends of vitamin E capsules and squeeze the contents into a teaspoonful of non-allergenic juice to get an infant to take the vitamin. There also are water-soluble fatty vitamin preparations for those with fibrocystic disease. Some children like the taste of vitamin E squirted directly onto their tongue, even in the most common oil form. Try whatever works: 100 IU per day is a good amount for most kids.

Even "vitamin E–rich" foods are not that rich: they might have just enough vitamin E to protect the long-chain fatty acids in them. A supplement form is needed. Vitamin E is safe and remarkably non-toxic. It provides the primary defense against the formation of dangerous lipid hydroperoxides (broken, oxidized fatty acids). For example, overexposure to oxygen has been a major cause of blindness in premature infants. Oxygen-tent retina damage is now prevented by giving "preemies" vitamin E, a natural antioxidant. The typical recommended dosage is 100 mg of vitamin E per kilogram body weight, which is around 200 IU for a preemie. This is equivalent to an adult dose of about 7,000 IU for an average-weight person. When you purchase vitamin E, be sure to get the natural form (d-alpha tocopherol) rather than the synthetic (d,l-alpha tocopherol) since it is much more efficient in preventing the formation of dangerous hydroperoxides. Here is a useful health tip: vitamin E applied to a scar, even a healed up "keloid," can bring about a disappearing act. Simply pierce both ends of a capsule, squeeze out a drop or two, and rub into the scar tissue daily. It takes a while, but watch and see the results.

Many doctors wrongly advise their patients that their children stand a chance of toxicity with megadoses. In fact, toxicity symptoms have not been reported even at intakes of 800 IU per kilogram of body weight daily for five months, according to the U.S. Food and Nutrition Board.[5] This demonstrated safe level would work out to around 56,000 IU daily for an average adult, some 5,000 times the RDA!

WHAT ABOUT IRON?

Iron is part of the make-up of hemoglobin and myoglobin ("heme," as in blood; "myo," as in muscle). These substances have the remarkable ability to grab onto or release oxygen and carbon dioxide at the right times and places. Anemia from iron deficiency is aptly called "iron-deficiency anemia," resulting in pallor and weakness. The anemia of children is due to either some subtle form of blood loss or inadequate intake of iron, either in elemental form or organic form. A simple look at red blood cells is diagnostic for iron-deficiency anemia. A little red meat and many vegetable sources, and the amount in a typical multivitamin/mineral preparation, do a good job of prevention. Giving vitamin C along with iron can enhance the correction of iron-deficiency anemia.

Minerals, which are chemically and nutritionally different from vitamins, have an excellent safety record, but not quite as good as vitamins. On the average, one or two fatalities per year are typically attributed to iron poisoning from gross overdosing on supplemental iron. Deaths attributed to other supplemental minerals are extremely rare. Even iron, although not as safe as vitamins, accounts for fewer deaths than do laundry and dishwashing detergents. Do not allow your child unfettered access to multivitamins containing iron (most iron-containing supplements have child-resistant caps as well). The amount of iron in multivitamins, even when taken twice daily, is fine. There were zero deaths in 2008–2009 from any mineral supplement, according to the U.S. National Poison Data System. This means there were no fatalities from calcium, magnesium, chromium, zinc, colloidal silver, selenium, iron, or multimineral supplements.

HOW TO GET KIDS TO TAKE THEIR VITAMINS

You cannot expect a small child to swallow a tablet or a chunk of a tablet. You can crush the tablet (or tablet fraction) and give the resulting powder in juice or mixed in a bit of food. Hot food is not an appropriate choice for heat-sensitive vitamins. Applesauce or other pureed fruit works well; pineapple or other sweet juice is fine, as well. Pick a food or drink that hides a vitamin taste nicely. Remember, you get to swallow these things whole. Vitamins are not put into tablets for nothing! I (AWS) still remember the time my father first gave me a vitamin pill when I was a kid. I innocently asked him if it was chewable or not and his answer was, "Try it." Crunch. Yuk.

Giving "doctored" portions early in the meal helps ensure children get down. Use as small an amount of juice or fruit as possible rather than "taint" an entire portion. The moment the dose is swallowed, immediately follow it with a favorite "chaser": sweet juice or fruit will take away any aftertaste. We would go so far as to have two cups of juice on the table in front of the child: one contained an eighth cup or less of juice with the powder mixed in; the other cup was comfortably full of juice only. The moment the odd-tasting juice disappeared, we had the yummy juice right at the kid's lips. Speed is important here. Hit the taste buds with a nice flavor before they even get a chance to figure out the first one.

Chewable supplements are tasty and convenient. Once a child is old enough to handle chewable tablets, he or she will usually take them without complaint. Beware of artificial colors, flavors, and especially sweeteners. These potentially harmful chemicals are money savers for the manufacturer and do no good for your child. Try a health food store, and always read labels.

Here is one way to tell if a child is old enough to swallow a vitamin tablet: offer a small cash reward if the kid can do it. Since chewable tablets tend to be more expensive than regular tablets containing the same amounts of nutrients, you will still be money ahead if this works. Start first with a small capsule. Tell the child that it is okay if they can't swallow this like a big boy or girl can. Pride and spending money seem to be an irresistible combination for kids. For the child of an age that should be able to handle a tablet or pill but says, "I can't swallow that monster," try this: have him or her put it under the tongue and not worry about it, then concentrate on swallowing a big gulp of water. The pill finds its way into the slipstream.

When in public places, keep supplements low-key. Likewise, when visiting relatives, there is no need to make a show or an issue over children's vitamins. You can give your child their vitamins before you leave home or when you get back. Chewable supplements that look and taste like candy are convenient in more ways than one. Health food stores and pharmacies have a variety of popular vitamin products that do not even resemble "pills." Technically, most schools require a letter from a doctor giving permission for a child to take supplements at school. If you can get such a letter from your doctor, it is handy to have. There is no reason for any kid to be singled out at school just because supplements have always been a part of their good diet. Most principals are sensitive to children's feelings and will respond well to your friendly parent note or phone call.

Your children don't like tablets? Many vitamins (notably vitamin C) are available in powdered form; some multiple vitamins are, too. If you cannot find powdered supplements, you can make your own: gelatin capsules may easily be pulled apart, and tablets can be crushed between two spoons or in a mortar and pestle. The result is utterly unflavored, so mix with juice or applesauce. Remember that the shelf life of liquid and powdered vitamins is much shorter than vitamins in capsules or tightly pressed tablets. We often put our vitamin C powder in small, easily closed bottles and work from them. Read expiration dates whenever you buy vitamins.

If too big to swallow, fat-soluble vitamins or fish oil that come in capsules should not be a problem. With a needle, poke a hole in each end and squeeze the contents into something tasty.

If a certain vitamin supplement does not agree with your child, you might want to simply try a different brand. Like ice cream, some products are artificially colored or flavored. Natural brands tend to be better in this regard. Always read the label, looking for what is not in the tablet as well as what is. It is worth remembering that many times a person is having a problem only with the tableting ingredients (excipients).

For brand suggestions, you might ask friends what ones they like and why. Health food stores are very willing to help you select an appropriate supplement. Health professionals may have an opinion as well. Remember to consider the source of your nutritional information. Let the buyer beware and do some research on the Internet. You need to know what you are doing, and why. Begin with *How to Live Longer and Feel Better* by Linus Pauling, who was an expert on vitamin supplementation. You can also write directly to manufacturers for a full disclosure of all ingredients and excipients in every nutritional product the company sells.

SAFETY OF NUTRITIONAL SUPPLEMENTS

There was not even one death caused by any dietary supplement in either 2008 or 2009, according to the most recent information collected by the U.S. National Poison Data System (NPDS). The annual report of the American Association of Poison Control Centers shows zero deaths from multiple vitamins; zero deaths from any of the B vitamins; zero deaths from vitamins A, C, D, or E; and zero deaths from any other vitamin.[6] Sixty poison centers provide coast-to-coast data for the NPDS, which is then reviewed by twenty-nine medical and clinical toxicologists.

Over half of the U.S. population takes daily nutritional supplements. Even if each of those people took only a single tablet daily, that makes 154,000,000 individual doses per day, for a total of over 56 billion doses annually. Since many persons take more than just one vitamin or mineral tablet, actual consumption is considerably higher, and the safety of nutritional supplements is all the more remarkable.

If nutritional supplements are allegedly so "dangerous," as the U.S. Food and Drug Administration and news media so often claim, then where are the bodies? Those who wonder if the media are biased against vitamins may consider this: how many television stations, newspapers, magazines, and medical journals have reported that no one dies from nutritional supplements? Consumers are not getting a fair picture of vitamin safety and efficacy from government-sponsored sources, particularly the National Institutes of Health. However, when they do have all the information, consumers see that vitamin supplements are far safer than drugs.[7]

Vitamin supplementation is not the problem. It is under-nutrition and over-medication that are the problems. Vitamins are the solution.

VITAMIN CONTROVERSY

"Vitamin-bashing" news media articles are typically based on studies with faulty design whose conclusions were preordained. One example is the meta-analysis, which is not new research but instead a review of existing research. It is not a clinical study, but rather a statistical look at a collection of studies. If you analyze enough failed studies, you will get a negative meta-analysis. If you exclude enough successful studies, you preordain the conclusion.

Proving Effectiveness

Low-dose vitamin studies are the ones that get negative results. Most vitamin research is low dose. You cannot test the effectiveness of high doses by giving low doses. Any time nutritional research employs inadequately low doses of vitamins—doses that hundreds of ortho-molecular physicians have already reported as too small to work—vitamin therapy will be touted as "ineffective." You can set up any study to fail. One way to ensure failure is to make a meaningless test, which is assured if you make the choice to use insufficient quantities of the substance to be investigated.

Proving Safety

One reason commonly offered to justify conducting low-dose studies is that high doses of vitamins are somehow dangerous. They are not. There are those who may not believe this next statement, but it is not a matter of belief—it is a matter of fact: there is not even one death per year from vitamin supplements. However, there are at least 106,000 deaths from drugs each year in the U.S., even when taken as prescribed. This may be a low estimate.

Abram Hoffer, M.D., Ph.D., who conducted the first double-blind, placebo-controlled studies in psychiatry, has called for similar stud-ies testing alleged vitamin side effects. He said, "Let the opponents of vitamin therapy cite the double-blind, placebo-controlled studies upon which they have based their toxicity allegations. They can't, because there aren't any."

Eliminating Bias

It is ironic that critics of vitamins preferentially cite low-dose studies in an attempt to show lack of vitamin effectiveness, yet they cannot cite any double-blind, placebo-controlled studies of high doses that show vitamin dangers. This is because vitamins are effective, and safe, at high doses. Health professionals and other interested persons are invited to personally search the literature for evidence of deaths caused by vitamin supplements—you will not find any.

SUMMARY

Decades ago, the mantra of the nutrition "experts" was "eat a *bal-*

anced diet." What foods were being balanced were inadequately described, but they were deemed sufficient. Extra vitamins were said to "just make expensive urine." Vitamins can do so much more than preventing deficiency diseases, which requires very low amounts. "Megadoses," used properly, can accomplish wonders. We have defined a healthy diet, which forms a base for health, but factors such as availability and cost may prohibit achieving it. While working toward that ideal, we also must fill in the gaps with supplementation of vitamins and other nutrients. The further away one is from eating a good diet, the greater the need for supplementation, not to substitute for but to augment. Nutritional supplements are safe and effective for children.

CONCLUSION

"Without health there is no happiness. An attention to health, then, should take the place of every other object."
—THOMAS JEFFERSON

In 1970, long hair was in, beads and blue jeans were what you'd wear, and there were protests everywhere. At the state college I (AWS) attended, everyone conformed by not conforming. Well, almost everyone—I met one person who was actually an individual. His family kept live rattlesnakes as pets, which initially seized my attention, but he proved to be the most interesting specimen in the house. A free-thinking but very short-haired fellow, who always wore an Oxford shirt and necktie to class, he described himself as a "militant middle of the roader." He was hard to pin down on any issue. He always insisted on reserving the right to decide for himself and simply did not care what others thought about him. He was too interested in the search for truth.

Now, over forty years later, I think I have a better idea of what he was on to. You have to make it happen yourself. Asking a physician to tell you what to do for your children may seem rather obvious, and attractively easy, but in the long run it will not work. If you would be a pilot, you have to hoist yourself into the left seat of an aircraft and take the time to learn to fly. If you are content to be a passenger in the medical system, you are reading the wrong book. If you want something done right, you have to do it yourself. This especially includes your health care: you can learn it, you can do it, and you can share the way with others.

Change your family's dietary lifestyle and you dramatically improve your health. "That's so simplistic!" rails our inner critic. We doubt natural therapy because it's too simple to work and we doubt self-care because we doubt ourselves. We've been educated to be good consumers, and that includes becoming consumers of health-care services. We have not been educated to be self-reliant.

The good news is that therapeutic nutrition is cheap, simple, effective, and safe. Of course, we have been taught that anything cheap, simple, and safe cannot possibly be effective against "real" diseases. And when, by our own verified experiences, we find that megavitamin therapy is cheap and effective, we have pharmaphilic fear-mongerers trying to tell us that it can't be safe.

Ultimately, we have to decide who we are going to listen to. I say, read the research for yourself and see for yourself. Everything changes the day you decide to no longer let your health-care providers treat you like a child. At first, it may not be easy to face down a domineering doctor or even to negotiate compromises with a family member. It is not easy to bring yourself to read the research, and it takes some gumption to try high-dose vitamin therapy for the first time.

Until you see how well it works, that is. And then, with experience, it becomes easier, like flying an airplane on instruments. The first time I (inadvertently) ended up inside a cloud, I had been naively trying to climb over it. A very low-time pilot, I had only a few short hours of instrument instruction. It immediately came in handy. The cloud was vastly bigger than I thought, and instead of my climbing over it, it climbed over me. The world instantly went white, and I could not see a thing. As if on a string, my head tilted down to the instrument panel and I could hear my ever-patient instructor's words playing back in my ear: "Look at the instruments. Wings straight and level. Fly the airplane." Those oh-so-very-elementary commands, by the way, can save your life. In what seemed like an eternity (but was actually only about half a minute), I flew out of the other side of the cloud into clear, blue sky again.

It gets easier all the time. I do not fear clouds; I just avoid them.

But next time I find myself in one, my experience will reconfirm what I'd taken the time to learn. Similarly, we do not need to fear illness— we need to learn what to do to avoid it and to fly out of it in one piece when it is suddenly upon us.

Behaviorist B.F. Skinner said that all learning is the mastery of a very large number of very small steps. And everybody knows the Chinese saying that the longest journey begins with a single step. Sure, asking another to do it for you is almost irresistibly easy. Learning to do it yourself isn't. But when you fly solo into one of life's many unscheduled but inevitable clouds, if you've practiced for it, you'll be ready.

Additional
Reading

Joseph Goldberger, M.D.

Alan Kraut's prize-winning book, *Goldberger's War: The Life and Work of a Public Health Crusader* (New York: Hill and Wang, 2003), is an excellent source on this outstanding pioneer.

Carlton Fredericks, Ph.D.

Fredericks, C. *Carlton Fredericks' New Low Blood Sugar and You.* New York: Perigee, 1985.

———. *Arthritis: Don't Learn to Live With It.* New York: Perigee, 1985.

———. *Carlton Fredericks' Program for Living Longer.* New York: Simon & Schuster, 1983.

———. *Carlton Fredericks' Nutrition Guide for the Prevention and Cure of Common Ailments and Diseases.* New York: Simon & Schuster, 1982.

———. *Dr. Carlton Fredericks' Low-Carbohydrate Diet.* New York: Award Books, 1965.

Lendon Smith, M.D.

Lendon Smith's bibliography is published online at: http://www.doctoryourself.com/biblio_lsmith.html.

Emanuel Cheraskin, M.D., D.M.D.

Dr. Cheraskin's complete bibliography of books and papers is posted online at: www.doctoryourself.com/biblio_cheraskin.html.

Claus W. Jungeblut, M.D.

Of Dr. Jungeblut's many research reports, twenty-two were published in the *Journal of Experimental Medicine*. They are archived and available online at: http://www.jem.org/ contents-by-date.0.shtml.

Key papers regarding ascorbate include:

Jungeblut, C.W. "Inactivation of Poliomyelitis Virus in Vitro by Crystalline Vitamin C (Ascorbic Acid)." *J Exp Med* 62 (October 1935): 517–521.

———. "Vitamin C Therapy and Prophylaxis in Experimental Poliomyelitis." *J Exp Med* 65 (1937): 127–146.

———. "Further Observations on Vitamin C Therapy in Experimental Poliomyelitis." *J Exp Med* 66 (1937): 459–477.

———. "A Further Contribution to Vitamin C Therapy in Experimental Poliomyelitis." *J Exp Med* 70 (1939): 315–332.

Jungeblut, C.W., and R.R. Feiner. "Vitamin C Content of Monkey Tissues in Experimental Poliomyelitis." *J Exp Med* 66 (1937): 479–491.

Benjamin F. Feingold, M.D.

Feingold, B.F. *Why Your Child is Hyperactive.* New York: Random House, 1985.

———. *Feingold Cookbook for Hyperactive Children.* New York: Random House, 1979.

———. *Introduction to Clinical Allergy.* Springfield, IL: Charles C. Thomas, 1973.

———. "The Role of Diet in Behavior." *Ecol Dis* 1:2–3 (1982): 153–165.

———. "Feingold Diet." *Aust Fam Physician* 9:1 (January 1980): 60–61.

———. "Dietary Management of Nystagmus." *J Neural Transm* 45:2 (1979): 107–115.

———. "Behavioral Disturbances Linked to the Ingestion of Food Additives." *Del Med J* 49:2 (February 1977): 89–94.

———. "Food Additives in Dentistry." *J Am Soc Prev Dent* 7:1 (January–February 1977): 13–15.

———. "Adverse Reactions to Food Additives with Special Reference to Hyperkinesis and Learning Difficulty (H-LD)." Monograph (1976), pp. 215–245.

———. "Hyperkinesis and Learning Disabilities Linked to Artificial Food Flavors and Colors." *Am J Nurs* 75:5 (May 1975): 797–780.

———. "Food Additives in Clinical Medicine." *Int J Dermatol* 14:2 (March 1975): 112–114.

———. "Letter: Biting Insects Survey: A Statistical Report." *Ann Allergy* 33:2 (August 1974): 128–129.

———. "Recognition of Food Additives as a Cause of Symptoms of Allergy." *Ann Allergy* 26:6 (June 1968): 309–313.

Freeman, E.H., F.J. Gorman, M.T. Singer, et al. "Personality Variables and Allergic Skin Reactivity. A Cross-validation Study." *Psychosom Med* 29:4 (June–August 1967): 312–322.

Michaeli, D., E. Benjamini, R.C. Miner, B.F. Feingold. "In Vitro Studies On the Role of Collagen in the Induction of Hypersensitivity to Flea Bites." *J Immunol* 97:3 (September 1966): 402–406.

Feingold, B.F., M.T. Singer, E.H. Freeman, A. Deskins. "Psychological Variables in Allergic Disease: A Critical Appraisal of Methodology." *J Allergy* 38:3 (September 1966): 143–155.

How to Improve a Child's Behavior Without Drugs

Canter, L. *Assertive Discipline for Parents*, Revised ed. New York: Harper and Row, 1985.

Cott, A., J. Agel, E. Boe. *Dr. Cott's Help for Your Learning Disabled Child: The Orthomolecular Treatment*. New York: Times Books, 1985.

Ginott, H.G. *Between Parent and Child*. New York: Morrow/Avon Books, 1976.

Hoffer, Abram. *Dr. Hoffer's ABC of Natural Nutrition for Children*. Kingston, Ontario, Canada: Quarry Press, 1999.

Phelan, Thomas W. *1-2-3 Magic: Effective Discipline for Children 2–12*. Glen Ellyn, IL: ParentMagic, 2010. (The video version by the same name is also highly recommended.)

Reed, Barbara. *Food, Teens and Behavior*. Manitowoc, WI: Natural Press, 1983.

Barbara and Paul Stitt

Reed, Barbara. *Food, Teens and Behavior*. Manitowoc, WI: Natural Press, 1983.

Stitt, Paul. *Fighting the Food Giants*, Revised ed. Manitowoc, WI: Natural Press, 1983.

William J. McCormick, M.D.

A review of Dr. McCormick's work, with bibliography: Saul, A.W. "Taking the Cure: The Pioneering Work of William J. McCormick, M.D." *J Orthomolecular Med* 18:2 (2003): 93-96. Available online at: http://www.doctoryourself.com/mccormick.html and http://orthomolecular.org/library/jom.

Frederick Robert Klenner, M.D.

Dr. Klenner's specific treatment protocols are described in: Smith, L.H. *Clinical Guide to the Use of Vitamin C: The Clinical Experiences of Frederick R. Klenner, M.D.* Portland, OR: Life Sciences Press, 1988. The full text of this book is posted online at: http://www.seanet.com/~alexs/ascorbate/198x/smith-lh-clinical_guide_1988.htm.

Biography and bibliography: Saul, A.W. "Hidden in Plain Sight: The Pioneering Work of Frederick Robert Klenner, M.D." *J Orthomolecular Med* 22:1 (2007): 31–38. Available online at: http://www.doctoryourself.com/klennerbio.html and http://orthomolecular.org/library/jom.

Robert F. Cathcart, M.D.

Dr. Cathcart's bibliography is available online at: http://www.doctoryourself.com/ biblio _cathcart.html.

Hugh D. Riordan, M.D.

Riordan, H.D., J.A. Jackson, M. Schultz, M. "Case Study: High-Dose Intravenous Vitamin C in the Treatment of a Patient with Adenocarcinoma of the Kidney." *J Orthomolecular Med* 5:1 (1990).

Jackson, J.A., H.D. Riordan, R.E. Hunninghake, N.H. Riordan. "High-dose Intravenous Vitamin C and Long-term Survival of a Patient with Cancer of Head of the Pancreas." *J Orthomolecular Med* 10:2 (1995).

Riordan, N.H., H.D. Riordan, X. Meng, et al. "Intravenous Ascorbate as a Tumor Cytotoxic Chemotherapeutic Agent." *Med Hypotheses* 44 (1995).

Riordan, N.H., J.A. Jackson, H.D. Riordan. "Intravenous Vitamin C in a Terminal Cancer Patient." *J Orthomolecular Med* 11:2 (1996).

Riordan, H.D., et al. "High-Dose Intravenous Vitamin C in the Treatment of a Patient with Renal Cell Carcinoma of the Kidney." *J Orthomolecular Med* 13:2 (1998).

Gonzalez, M.J., E. Mora, N.H. Riordan, et al. "Rethinking Vitamin C and Cancer: An Update on Nutritional Oncology." *Cancer Prevent Int* 3 (1998): 215–224.

Gonzalez, M.J., E.M. Mora, J.R. Miranda-Massari, et al. "Inhibition of Human Breast Carcinoma Cell Proliferation by Ascorbate and Copper." *P R Health Sci J* 21:1 (March 2002).

Gonzalez, M.J., J.R. Miranda-Massari, E.M. Mora, et al. "Orthomolecular Oncology: a Mechanistic View of Intravenous Ascorbate's Chemotherapeutic Activity." *P R Health Sci J* 21:1 (March 2002).

Riordan, H.D., R.E. Hunninghake, N.H. Riordan, et al. "Intravenous Ascorbic Acid: Protocol for its Application and Use." *P R Health Sci* J 22:3 (September 2003).

Padayatty, S.J., H. Sun, Y. Wang, et al. "Vitamin C Pharmacokinetics: Implications for Oral and Intravenous Use." *Ann Intern Med* 140:7 (April 2004): 533–537.

Riordan, H.D., N.H. Riordan, J.A. Jackson, et al. "Intravenous Vitamin C as a Chemotherapy Agent: a Report on Clinical Cases." *P R Health Sci J* 23:2 (June 2004): 115–118.

Dr. Riordan's bibliography is available at: http://www.doctoryourself.com/biblio_riordan.html.

Mercury Amalgam Fillings

Additional information on the health effects of mercury is available from the U.S. Environmental Protection Agency's IRIS database at: http://www.epa.gov/iris/subst/0370.htm.

Information on the Mercury Controversy from Norway: press release: http://www.regjeringen.no/en/dep/md/press-centre/Press-releases/2007/Bans-mercury-in-products.html?id=495138; regulation: http://www.regjeringen.no/Upload/MD/Vedlegg/Forskrifter/product_regulation_amendment_071214.pdf.

Information on the Mercury Controversy from Denmark: http://nyhederne.tv2 .dk/article.php/id-9868029.html and http://www.dr.dk/Nyheder/Indland/2007/12/ 31/174314.htm?nyheder.

Information on the Mercury Controversy from Sweden: http://www.dn.se/DNet/ jsp/polopoly.jsp?d=147&a=728814 and http://www.svd.se/nyheter/inrikes/artikel _724369.svd.

Information on the Mercury Controversy from Canada: http://www.hc-sc.gc.ca/dhp-mps/md-im/applic-demande/pubs/dent_amalgam-eng.php.

Information on the Mercury Controversy from France: http://afssaps.sante.fr/ ang/pdf/amalgam.pdf.

Review and commentary: http://www.yourhealthbase.com/amalgams.html and http://www.mercurypolicy.org.

Video on amalgam fillings: http://www.foodmatters.tv/mercury-madness.html video by the International Academy of Oral Medicine and Toxicology (http:// www.iaomt.org/); available for viewing on YouTube: http://www.youtube.com/ watch?v=9ylnQ-T7oiA.

Vitamin D

[No authors listed.] "Vitamin D—Monograph." *Altern Med Rev* 13:2 (June 2008): 153–164. http://www.thorne.com/altmedrev/.fulltext/13/2/153.pdf.

Cannell, J.J., and B.W. Hollis. "Use of Vitamin D in Clinical Practice." *Altern Med Rev* 13:1 (March 2008): 6–20. http://www.thorne.com/altmedrev/.fulltext/13/1/6.pdf.

Dietrich, T., K.J. Joshipura, B. Dawson-Hughes, H.A. Bischoff-Ferrari. "Association Between Serum Concentrations of 25-Hydroxyvitamin D_3 and Periodontal Disease in the U.S. Population." *Am J Clin Nutr* 80:1 (July 2004): 108–113. http://www.ajcn.org/cgi/reprint/80/1/108

Dunning, J.M. "The Influence of Latitude and Distance from Seacoast on Dental Disease." *J Dent Res* 32:6 (December 1953): 811–829. http://jdr.sagepub.com/ cgi/reprint/32/6/811.

East, B.R. "Mean annual hours of sunshine and the incidence of dental caries." Am J Public Health Nations Health 29:7 (July 1939): 777-780. http://www .ajph.org/cgi/reprint/29/7/777.

Garland, C.F., F.C. Garland, E.D. Gorham, et al. "The Role of Vitamin D in Cancer Prevention." *Am J Public Health* 96:2 (February 2006): 252–261. http://www.ajph.org/cgi/reprint/96/2/252.

Grant, W.B. "In Defense of the Sun: An Estimate of Changes in Mortality Rates in the United States If Mean Serum 25-Hydroxyvitamin D Levels Were Raised to

45 ng/mL by Solar Ultraviolet-B Irradiance." *Dermato-Endocrinology* 1:4 (2009): 207–214.   http://www.landesbioscience.com/journals/dermatoendocrinology/ archive/volume/1/issue/4/.

Holick, M.F. "Vitamin D Deficiency." *N Engl J Med* 357:3 (2007): 266–281. http://content.nejm.org/cgi/content/short/357/3/266.

Martins, D., M. Wolf, D. Pan, et al. "Prevalence of Cardiovascular Risk Factors and the Serum Levels of 25-Hydroxyvitamin D in the United States: Data from the Third National Health and Nutrition Examination Survey." *Arch Intern Med* 167:11 (2007): 1159–1165. http://archinte.ama-assn.org/cgi/reprint/167/11/1159.

Melamed, M.L., E.D. Michos, W. Post, B. Astor. "25-Hydroxyvitamin D Levels and the Risk of Mortality in the General Population." *Arch Intern Med* 168:15 (2008): 1629–1637. http://archinte.ama-assn.org/cgi/reprint/168/15/1629.

Papandreou, D., P. Malindretos, Z. Karabouta, I. Rousso. "Possible Health Implications and Low Vitamin D Status during Childhood and Adolescence: An Updated Mini Review." *Int J Endocrinol* 2010 (2010): Article 472173. http://www .ncbi.nlm.nih.gov/pmc/articles/PMC2778445/pdf/IJE2010-472173.pdf.

Wang, T.J., M.J. Pencina, S.L. Booth, et al. "Vitamin D Deficiency and Risk of Cardiovascular Disease." Circulation 117:4 (January 2008): 503–511. http://circ .ahajournals.org/cgi/content/full/117/4/503.

REFERENCES

Chapter 1: Discovering the Power of Vitamins and Other Nutrients

1. Elmore, J.G., and A.R. Feinstein. "Joseph Goldberger: An Unsung Hero of American Clinical Epidemiology." *Ann Intern Med* 121:5 (September 1994): 372–375.

2. Hoffer, Abram. Personal communication with AWS.

3. Nathoo, T., C.P. Holmes, A. Ostry. "An Analysis of the Development of Canadian Food Fortification Policies: The Case of Vitamin B." *Health Promot Int* 20:4 (2005): 375–382.

4. Office of NIH History. "Dr. Joseph Goldberger and the War on Pellagra." Bethesda, MD: National Institutes of Health. http://history.nih.gov/exhibits/goldberger/index.html. Accessed January 2011.

5. Pollan, Michael. *In Defense of Food.* New York: Penguin, 2008.

6. Dickey, L.D. (ed.). *Clinical Ecology.* Springfield, IL: Charles C. Thomas, 1976.

7. Smith, Lendon. *Feed Yourself Right.* New York: McGraw, 1983, xiii–xiv.

8. Ibid., p. 61.

9. Adapted from an article in the *Journal of Orthomolecular Medicine* 16:4 (2001): 248–250. Used with permission.

Chapter 2: Go to the Doctor or Become the Doctor?

1. Nearing, Scott. *The Making of a Radical,* 2nd ed. Harborside, ME: Social Science Institute, 1976, p. 222.

Chapter 3: The Truth About Antibiotics and Immunizations

1. Lyman, Howard F., with Glen Merzer. *Mad Cowboy: Plain Truth from the Cattle Rancher Who Won't Eat Meat.* New York: Scribner, 1998.

2. Hergenrather, J., G. Hlady, B. Wallace, E. Savage. "Pollutants in Breast Milk of Vegetarians." *New Engl J Med* 304:13 (March 1981): 792.

3. Kenny, A. "Whooping Cough Cases Spread." *New York Times* (October 26, 2003).

4. New York State Department of Health. "Immunization." http://www.health .state.ny.us/nysdoh/immun/pdf/2378.pdf.

5. The Vitamin D Council. http://www.vitamindcouncil.org. Cannell, J.J., et al. "Epidemic Influenza and Vitamin D." *Epidemiol Infect* 134:6 (December 2006): 1129–1140. Available online at: http://www.biochem.wisc.edu/courses/biochem 901/secure/materials/ readings/09_Cannell.pdf.

6. Tavera-Mendoza, L.E., and J.H. White. "Cell Defenses and the sunshine vitamin." Sci Am (November 2007): 62–72.

7. Kaiser, J.D., et al. "Micronutrient Supplementation Increases CD4 Count in HIV-infected Individuals on Highly Active Antiretroviral Therapy: A Prospective, Double-blinded, Placebo-controlled Trial." *J Acquired Immune Deficiency Syn* 42:5 (2006): 523–528.

8. UNICEF. "State of the World's Children 1998." Figure 11: Measles deaths and vitamin A supplementation. Available online at: http://www.unicef.org/sowc98/ fig11.htm.

9. Jungeblut, C.W. "Inactivation of Poliomyelitis Virus by Crystallin Vitamin C (Ascorbic Acid)." *J Exp Med* 62 (1935): 517–521.

10. Miller, N.Z. "Vaccines and Natural Health." *Mothering* (Spring 1994): 44–54.

11. The Advisory Committee on Immunization Practices. "Notice to Readers: Recommended Childhood Immunization Schedule—United States, 2000." *MMWR* 49:02 (January 2000): 35–38, 47.

12. Jungeblut, C.W. "Inactivation of Poliomyelitis Virus by Crystallin Vitamin C (Ascorbic Acid)." *J Exp Med* 62 (1935): 517–521.

13. Jungeblut, C.W., and R.L. Zwemer. "Inactivation of Diphtheria Toxin in Vivo and in Vitro by Crystalline Vitamin C (Ascorbic Acid)." *Proc Soc Exp Biol Med* 32 (1935): 1229–1234. Jungeblut, C.W. "Inactivation of Tetanus Toxin by Crystalline Vitamin C (L-Ascorbic Acid)." *J Immunol* 33 (1937): 203–214.

14. "Polio Clues." *Time* (September 18, 1939).

15. Stone, I. "Viral Infection." *The Healing Factor,* Chapter 13. New York: Grosset and Dunlap, 1972. This book is posted online at: http://vitamincfoundation .org/stone/.

16. Klenner, F.R. "The Use of Vitamin C as an Antibiotic." *J Appl Nutr* 6 (1953): 274–278.

17. Klenner, F.R. "The Treatment of Poliomyelitis and Other Virus Diseases with Vitamin C." *South Med Surg* (July 1949): 209.

18. Chor, J.S.Y., K.L.K. Ngai, W.B. Goggins, et al. "Willingness of Hong Kong Healthcare Workers to Accept Pre-pandemic Influenza Vaccination at Different WHO Alert Levels: Two Questionnaire Surveys." *Br Med J* 339 (2009): b3391. http://www.bmj.com/cgi/content/abstract/339/aug25_2/b3391.

CHAPTER 267

19. Fox News. Foxnews.com. http://www.foxnews.com/opinion/2009/08/26/think-greater-risk/.

20. Burch, J., M. Corbett, C. Stock, et al. "Prescription of Anti-influenza Drugs for Healthy Adults: A Systematic Review and Meta-analysis." *The Lancet Infect Dis* 9:9 (2009): 537–545. http://www.thelancet.com/journals/laninf/article/PIIS1473-3099(09)70199-9/fulltext.

21. Mercola, J. "Swine Flu Vaccine Makers to Profit $50 Billion a Year!!" Mercola.com. http://articles.mercola.com/sites/articles/archive/2009/08/13/Swine-Flu-Vaccine-Makers-to-Profit-50-Billion-a-Year.aspx.

22. Simonsen, L., T.A. Reichert, et al. "Impact of Influenza Vaccination on Seasonal Mortality in the U.S. Elderly Population." *Arch Intern Med* 165 (2005): 265–272.

23. Alliance for Natural Health. http://www.anhcampaign.org/.

24. Zimmer, S.M., and D.S. Burke. "Historical Perspective—Emergence of Influenza A (H1N1) Viruses." *N Engl J Med* 361 (2009): 279–285. http://content.nejm.org/cgi/content/full/361/3/279.

Chapter 4: How to Boost Your Child's Immune System Without Booster Shots

1. Cheraskin, E. "The Health of the Naturopath: Vitamin Supplementation and Psychologic State." *J Orthomolecular Med* 13 (4th Quarter 1998). Chandra, R.K. "Effect of Vitamin and Trace-element Supplementation on Immune Responses and Infection in Elderly Subjects." *The Lancet* 340:8828 (1992): 1124–1127. Pike, J., and R.K. Chandra. "Effect of Vitamin and Trace Element Supplementation on Immune Indices in Healthy Elderly." *Int J Vitam Nutr Res* 65:2 (1995): 117–120.

2. Dr. Cheraskin's complete bibliography of books and papers is posted online at: http://www.doctoryourself.com/biblio_cheraskin.html.

3. Meydani, S.N., M.P. Barklund, S. Liu, et al. "Effect of Vitamin E Supplementation on Immune Responsiveness of Healthy Elderly Subjects." *FASEB J* 3 (1989): A1057. Meydani, S.N., M.P. Barklund, S. Liu, et al. "Vitamin E Supplementation Enhances Cell-mediated Immunity in Healthy Elderly Subjects." *Am J Clin Nutr* 52:3 (September 1990): 557–563. See also: Cheraskin, E. "Antioxidants in Health and Disease: The Big Picture." *J Orthomolecular Med* 10:2 (Second Quarter 1995): 89–96.

4. Alexander, M., H. Newmark, R.G. Miller. "Oral Beta Carotene Can Increase the Number of OKT4+ Cells in Human Blood." *Immunol Lett* 9 (1985): 221–224.

5. Graham, N. *Am J Epidemiol* (December 1993).

6. Berkow, R. (ed.). *Merck Manual*, 14th ed. Whitehouse Station, NJ: Merck, 1982, p. 891.

7. Alpert, H.R., I. Behm, G.N. Connolly, Z. Kabir. "Smoke-free Households with

Children and Decreasing Rates of Paediatric Clinical Encounters for Otitis Media in the United States." *Tobacco Control* (January 26, 2011).

Chapter 5: What is the Healthiest Diet for Your Child?

1. Donini, L.M., D. Marsili, M.P. Graziani, et al. "Orthorexia Nervosa: A Preliminary Study with a Proposal for Diagnosis and an Attempt to Measure the Dimension of the Phenomenon." *Eat Weight Disord* 9:2 (June 2004): 151–157.

2. *The Observer* (August 16, 2009): 12. http://www.guardian.co.uk/society/2009/aug/16/orthorexia-mental-health-eating-disorder.

3. U.S. Food and Drug Administration. http://www.fda.gov/.

4 Cornell University Division of Nutritional Sciences. http://www.nutrition.cornell.edu/ChinaProject/results.html.

5. Price, W.A. *Nutrition and Physical Degeneration,* 8th ed. La Mesa, CA: Price-Pottenger Nutrition Foundation, 2008, p. 44.

6. Ibid.

7. Williams, S. *Nutrition and Diet Therapy,* 7th ed. St. Louis: Mosby, 1993.

8. TBS Network. Earth (February 4, 1996).

9. Farrell, W. *The Myth of Male Power.* New York: Berkley, 2001, p 109.

10. National Hot Dog & Sausage Council. http://www.hot-dog.org.

11. Peters, J.M., S. Preston-Martin, S.J. London, et al. "Processed Meats and Risk of Childhood Leukemia." *Cancer Causes Control* 5:2 (March 1994): 195–202.

12. Nothlings, U., L.R. Wilkens, S.P. Murphy, et al. "Meat and Fat Intake as Risk Factors for Pancreatic Cancer: The Multiethnic Cohort Study." *J Natl Cancer Inst* 97 (2005): 1458–1465.

13. Sarasua, S., and D.A. Savitz. "Cured and Broiled Meat Consumption in Relation to Childhood Cancer: Denver, Colorado (United States)." *Cancer Causes Control* 5:2 (March 1994): 141–148.

14. Scanlan, R.A. "Nitrosamines and Cancer." The Linus Pauling Institute. http://lpi.oregonstate.edu/f-w00/nitrosamine.html. Cass, H., and J. English. *User's Guide to Vitamin C.* Laguna Beach, CA: Basic Health, 2002, pp. 64–67.

15. *Dr. Julian Whitaker's Health & Healing* 8:10 (October 1998).

16. DoctorYourself.com. "Effectively Managing a Child's Behavior" http://www.doctoryourself.com/kidraise.html and "Food, Thought, and Behavior" http://www.doctoryourself.com/hoffer_imbalance.html.

Chapter 6: Children and Cholesterol

1. National Center for Chronic Disease Prevention and Health Promotion, U.S. Centers for Disease Control and Prevention. "Childhood Obesity." http://www.cdc.gov/HealthyYouth/obesity/.

2. Ornish, D. *Newsweek* (May 27, 2008). http://www.newsweek.com/id/138837.

CHAPTER 269

3. Tanner, L. "Cholesterol Drugs Recommended for Some 8-Year-Olds." Associated Press.

4. "Cholesterol-Lowering Drugs for Eight-Year-Old Kids? American Academy of Pediatrics Urging 'McMedicine'." Orthomolecular Medicine News Service (August 18, 2008).

5. American Academy of Pediatrics. "Friends of Children Fund Corporate Members." http://www.aap.org/donate/FCFhonorroll.HTM.

6. Williams, R. *Nutrition Against Disease.* New York: Bantam, 1981.

7. Pollan, Michael. *In Defense of Food.* New York: Penguin, 2008.

8. Willett, W.C. "Trans Fatty Acids and Cardiovascular Disease—Epidemiological Data." *Atherosclerosis Suppl* 7:2 (May 2006): 5–8.

Chapter 7: A Toxic Environment and What To Do About It

1. Ho, M-W., and J. Cummins. "Glyphosate Toxic and Roundup Worse." Institute for Science in Society (March 7, 2005). http://www.i-sis.org.uk/GTARW.php.

2. Ibid.

3. Ibid.

4 Scheele, J., M. Teufel, K.H. Niessen. "Chlorinated Hydrocarbons in the Bone Marrow of Children: Studies on Their Association with Leukaemia." *Eur J Pediatr* 151:11 (1992): 802–805.

5. Ascherio, A., H. Chen, M.G. Weisskopf, et al. "Pesticide Exposure and Risk for Parkinson's Disease." *Ann Neurol* 60:2 (August 2006): 197–203. See also: Gatto, N.M., M. Cockburn, J. Bronstein, et al. "Well-water Consumption and Parkinson's Disease in Rural California." *Environ Health Perspect* 117:12 (December 2009): 1912–1918. Manthripragada, A.D., S. Costello, M.G. Cockburn, et al. "Paraoxonase 1, Agricultural Organophosphate Exposure, and Parkinson Disease." *Epidemiology* 21:1 (January 2010): 87–94. Kamel, F., and J.A. Hoppin. "Association of Pesticide Exposure with Neurologic Dysfunction and Disease." *Environ Health Perspect* 2004 112:9 (June 2004): 950–958. Arima, H., K. Sobue, M. So, et al. "Transient and Reversible Parkinsonism After Acute Organophosphate Poisoning." *J Toxicol Clin Toxicol* 41:1 (2003): 67–70. Bhatt, M.H., M.A. Elias, A.K. Mankodi. "Acute and Reversible Parkinsonism Due to Organophosphate Pesticide Intoxication: Five Cases." *Neurology* 52:7 (April 1999): 1467–1471. Müller-Vahl, K.R., H. Kolbe, R. Dengler. "Transient Severe Parkinsonism After Acute Organophosphate Poisoning." *J Neurol Neurosurg Psychiatry* 66:2 (February 1999): 253–254.

6. Hayden, K.M., M.C. Norton, D. Darcey, et al. "Occupational Exposure to Pesticides Increases the Risk of Incident AD: The Cache County Study." *Neurology* 74:19 (May 2010): 1524–1530.

7. Bouchard, M.F., D.C. Bellinger, R.O. Wright, M.G. Weisskopf. "Attention-deficit/Hyperactivity Disorder and Urinary Metabolites of Organophosphate Pesticides." *Pediatrics* 125:6 (June 2010): e1270–e1277.

8. Fialka, J.J. "EPA Scientists Cite Pressure In Pesticide Study: Union Files Letter Blasting Agency Managers, Industry Over Tests on Toxics Family." *Wall Street Journal* (May 25, 2006): A4.

9. Ames, B., F. Lee, W. Durston. "An Improved Bacterial Test System for the Detection and Classification of Mutagens and Carcinogens." *Proc Natl Acad Sci USA* 70 (1973): 782–786. See also: Mortelmans, K., and E. Zeiger. "The Ames Salmonella/Microsome Mutagenicity Assay." *Mutat Res* 455 (2000): 29–60.

10. Geier DA, Sykes LK, Geier MR. A Review of Thimerosal (Merthiolate) and its Ethylmercury Breakdown Product: Specific Historical Considerations Regarding Safety and Effectiveness. *Journal of Toxicology and Environmental Health*, Part B, 10:575–596, 2007.

11. American Academy of Pediatrics. *Pediatric Nutrition Handbook*. Evanston, IL: AAP, 1999.

12. U.S. Consumer Product Safety Commission (CPSC). Download report at: http://www.cpsc.gov/cpscpub/prerel/prhtml03/03004.pdf.

13. "Mercury Dental Amalgams Banned in 3 Countries: FDA, EPA, ADA Still Allow and Encourage Heavy-Metal Fillings." Orthomolecular Medicine News Service (November 20, 2008); http://orthomolecular.org/resources/omns/v04n24 .shtml.

14. Lowes, R. "FDA Hearing on Mercury-Based Dental Fillings Pleases Both Sides of Debate." *Medscape Medical News* (December 18, 2010).

15. Ibid.

16. "Dental Mercury Use Banned in Norway, Sweden and Denmark." Reuters (January 3, 2008); http://www.reuters.com/article/pressRelease/idUS108558+03-Jan-2008+PRN20080103.

17. Borane, V.R., and S.P. Zambare. "Role of Ascorbic Acid in Lead and Cadmium Induced Changes on the Blood Glucose Level of the Freshwater Fish, *Channa orientalis.*" *J Aquatic Biol* 21:2 (2006): 244–248. Gajawat, S., G. Sancheti, P.K. Goyal. "Vitamin C Against Concomitant Exposure to Heavy Metal and Radiation: A Study on Variations in Hepatic Cellular Counts." *Asian J Exp Sci* 19:2 (2005): 53–58. Shousha, W.G. "The Curative and Protective Effects of L-Ascorbic Acid and Zinc Sulphate on Thyroid Dysfunction and Lipid Peroxidation in Cadmium-intoxicated Rats." *Egypt J Biochem Mol Biol* 22:1 (2004): 1–16. Vasiljeva, S., N. Berzina, I. Remeza. "Changes in Chicken Immunity Induced by Cadmium, and the Protective Effect of Ascorbic Acid." *Proc Latvian Acad Sci Sect B: Natural Exact Appl Sci* 57:6 (2003): 232–237. Mahajan, A.Y., and S.P. Zambare. "Ascorbate Effect on Copper Sulphate and Mercuric Chloride Induced Alterations of Protein Levels in Freshwater Bivalve *Corbicula striatella.*" *Asian J Microbiol Biotech Environ Sci* 3:1–2 (2001): 95–100. Norwood, Jr., J., A.D. Ledbetter, D.L. Doerfler, et al. "Residual Oil Fly Ash Inhalation in Guinea Pigs: Influence of Ascorbate and Glutathione Depletion." *Toxicol Sci* 61:1 (2001): 144–153. Guillot, I., P. Bernard, W.A. Rambeck. "Influence of Vitamin C on the Retention of Cadmium in Turkeys." Vitamine und Zusatzstoffe in der Ernaehrung von Mensch und Tier, 5th Symposium, September 28–29, 1995, Jena, pp. 233–237.

CHAPTER 271

18. "Vitamin Supplements Help Protect Children from Heavy Metals, Reduce Behavioral Disorders." Orthomolecular Medicine News Service (October 8, 2007); http://orthomolecular.org/resources/omns/v03n07.shtml.

19. "EPA Study on Nickel Releases from Burning Coal." Download at: http://www.epa.gov/ttn/chief/le/nickel.pdf. The study shows about 10 percent of nickel in coal is released into the air. The press release estimates 10 percent of the other metals in coal with similar properties to nickel are also released into the air.

20. "Vitamin Supplements Help Protect Children from Heavy Metals, Reduce Behavioral Disorders." Orthomolecular Medicine News Service (October 8, 2007); http://orthomolecular.org/resources/omns/v03n07.shtml.

21. Lewinska, A., and G. Bartosz. "Protection of Yeast Lacking the Ure2 Protein Against the Toxicity of Heavy Metals and Hydroperoxides by Antioxidants." *Free Radical Res* 41:5 (2007): 580–590.

22. Saul, A.W. "Vitamins and Food Supplements: Safe and Effective." Testimony before the Government of Canada, 38th Parliament, 1st Session, Standing Committee on Health. Ottawa, Ontario, Canada, May 12, 2005; http://www.doctoryourself.com/testimony.htm.

23. U.S. Food and Drug Administration. "Update on Bisphenol A for Use in Food Contact Applications: January 2010." http://www.fda.gov/newsevents/publichealthfocus/ucm197739.htm.

24. Braun, J.M., K. Yolton, K.N. Dietrich, et al. "Prenatal Bisphenol A Exposure and Early Childhood Behavior." *Environ Health Perspect* 117:12 (December 2009): 1945–1952. See also: Braun, J.M., and R. Hauser. "Bisphenol A and Children's Health." *Curr Opin Pediatr* (February 2011).

25. Veurink, M., M. Koster, L.T. Berg. "The History of DES, Lessons to Be Learned." *Pharm World Sci* 27:3 (June 2005): 139–143. Tedeschi, C.A., M. Rubin, B.A. Krumholz. "Six Cases of Women with Diethylstilbestrol in Utero Demonstrating Long-term Manifestations and Current Evaluation Guidelines." *J Low Genit Tract Dis* 9:1 (January 2005): 11–18. Titus-Ernstoff, L., R. Troisi, E.E. Hatch, et al. "Offspring of Women Exposed in Utero to Diethylstilbestrol (DES): A Preliminary Report of Benign and Malignant Pathology in the Third Generation. " *Epidemiology* 19:2 (March 2008): 251–257.

26. Panzica, G., E. Mura, M. Pessatti, C. Viglietti-Panzica. "Early Embryonic Administration of Xenoestrogens Alters Vasotocin System and Male Sexual Behavior of the Japanese Quail." *Domest Anim Endocrinol* 29:2 (August 2005): 436–445.

27. Beltrán-Aguilar, E.D., L. Barker, B.A. Dye. Prevalence and Severity of Dental Fluorosis in the United States, 1999–2004. NCHS Data Brief, No. 53. Bethesda, MD: U.S. Centers for Disease Control and Prevention, National Center for Health Statistics, November 2010, p. 1.

28. Samuel J. Forman. *Infant Nutrition.* St. Louis: W.B. Saunders, 2nd edition, 1974.

29. American Academy of Pediatrics. *Pediatric Nutrition Handbook.* Evanston, IL: AAP, 1999.

30. Beltrán-Aguilar, E.D., L. Barker, B.A. Dye. Prevalence and Severity of Dental Fluorosis in the United States, 1999–2004. NCHS Data Brief, No. 53. Bethesda, MD: U.S. Centers for Disease Control and Prevention, National Center for Health Statistics, November 2010, p. 1.

Chapter 8: Obesity and Diabetes

1. "Modern Marvels: The Quest for Health," A&E TV, 1998.

2. *USA Today,* May 31, 2000.

3. http://www.iht.com/articles/72321.html

4. Center for Science in the Public Interest. "Liquid Candy." http://www .cspinet.org/liquidcandy/index.html.

5. Atkins, Robert C. *Atkins for Life.* New York: St. Martin's Press, 2003.

Chapter 9: Allergies and Asthma

1. Sears, Barry. *The Zone.* New York: HarperCollins, 1995

2. Bookman, R. "101 Hints, Tips and Bits of Wisdom from the President's Allergist: Timely Help for People with Allergies and Asthma." *Rodale's Allergy Relief* 3:7 (July 1988): 1–8. See also: Bookman, R. *The Dimensions of Clinical Allergy.* Springfield, IL: Charles C. Thomas, 1985.

3. Hatch, G.E. *Am J Clin Nutr* 61 (1995): 625S–630S.

4. Cathcart, R.F. "Vitamin C, Titrating to Bowel Tolerance, Anascorbemia, and Acute Induced Scurvy." *Med Hypotheses* 7 (1981): 1359–1376; http://www.doctoryourself.com/titration.html.

5. "Allergies." DoctorYourself.com. http://doctoryourself.com/allergies.html. See: Stone, I. *The Healing Factor.* New York: Grosset and Dunlap, 1972. The complete text of this book is posted online at: http://vitamincfoundation.org/stone/. Also see: "Asthma." CforYourself.com. http://www.cforyourself.com/Conditions/Asthma/asthma.html.

6. Ahluwalia, S.K., and E.C. Matsui. "The Indoor Environment and Its Effects on Childhood Asthma." *Curr Opin Allergy Clin Immunol* 11:2 (April 2011): 137–143. Kabir, Z., and L. Clancy. "Second-Hand Tobacco Smoke and Allergens—Double Jeopardy for Childhood Asthma Exacerbations." *Respiration* 81:3 (2011): 177–178. Mackay, D., S. Haw, J.G. Ayres, et al. "Smoke-free Legislation and Hospitalizations for Childhood Asthma." *N Engl J Med* 363:12 (September 2010): 1139–1145.

7. Cohen, R.T., B.A. Raby, K. Van Steen, et al.; Childhood Asthma Management Program Research Group. "In Utero Smoke Exposure and Impaired Response to Inhaled Corticosteroids in Children with Asthma." *J Allergy Clin Immunol* 126:3 (September 2010): 491–497.

8. Honsberger, R.W., and A.F. Wilson. "The Effect of Transcendental Meditation

Upon Bronchial Asthma." *Clin Res* 21 (1973): 278 (Abstract). Honsberger, R.W., and A.F. Wilson. "Transcendental Meditation in Treating Asthma." *Resp Ther J Inhalat Tech* 3 (1973): 79–80. Wilson, A.F., R.W. Honsberger, J.T. Chiu, H.S. Novey. "Transcendental Meditation and Asthma." *Respiration* 32 (1975): 74–80.

9. Graf, D., and G. Pfisterer. "Der Nutzen der Technik der Transzendentalen Meditation für die ärztliche Praxis." *Erfahrungsheilkunde* 9 (1978): 594–596. Kirtane, L. "Transcendental Meditation: A Multipurpose Tool in Clinical Practice." General medical practice, Poona, Maharashtra, India (1980). Browne, G.E., D. Fougere, A. Roxburgh, et al. "Improved Mental and Physical Health and Decreased Use of Prescribed and Non-prescribed Drugs Through the Transcendental Meditation Program." Age of Enlightenment Medical Council, Christchurch, New Zealand; Heylen Research Centre, Auckland, New Zealand; and Dunedin Hospital, Dunedin, New Zealand (1983).

10. Baker, J.C., and J.G. Ayres. "Diet and Asthma." *Resp Med* 94 (2000): 925–934.

11. Gazdik, F., M.R. Pijak, K. Gazdikova. "Need of Complementary Therapy With Selenium in Asthmatics." *Nutrition* 20:10 (2004): 950–952.

Chapter 10: Attention-Deficit Hyperactivity Disorder (ADHD)

1. Nair, J., U. Ehimare, B.D. Beitman, et al. "Clinical Review: Evidence-based Diagnosis and Treatment of ADHD in Children." *Mo Med* 103:6 (2006): 617–621. Rader, R., L. McCauley, E.C. Callen. "Current Strategies in the Diagnosis and Treatment of Childhood Attention-deficit/Hyperactivity Disorder." *Am Fam Physician* 79:8 (April 2009): 657–665. Singh, I. "Beyond Polemics: Science and Ethics of ADHD." *Nature Rev Neurosci* 9:12 (December 2008): 957–964.

2. American Academy of Pediatrics. "Clinical Practice Guideline: Diagnosis and Evaluation of the Child With Attention-Deficit/Hyperactivity Disorder. Committee on Quality Improvement, Subcommittee on Attention-Deficit/Hyperactivity Disorder." *Pediatrics* 105:5 (May 2000): 1158–1170.

3. DSM-IV-TR Workgroup. *The Diagnostic and Statistical Manual of Mental Disorders*, 4th edition, Text Revision. Washington, DC: American Psychiatric Association, 2000.

4. National Institutes of Health. *Attention Deficit Hyperactivity Disorder (ADHD)*. NIH Publication No. 08-3572. Bethesda, MD: U.S. Department of Health and Human Services, NIH, 2008.

5. Bailly, L. "Stimulant Medication for the Treatment of Attention-deficit Hyperactivity Disorder: Evidence-b(i)ased Practice?" *Psychiatric Bull (Royal Coll Psychiatry)* 29:8 (2005): 284–287.

6. NYU Child Study Center. About Our Kids. http://www.aboutourkids.org.

7. Jones, T.W., W.P. Borg, S.D. Boulware, et al. "Enhanced Adrenomedullary Response and Increased Susceptibility to Neuroglycopenia: Mechanisms Underlying the Adverse Effects of Sugar Ingestion in Healthy Children." *J Pediatr* 126:2 (February 1995): 171–177.

8. Roy, A., M. Virkkunen, M. Linnoila. "Monoamines, Glucose Metabolism, Aggression Towards Self and Others." *Int J Neurosci* 41:3–4 (August 1988): 261–264.

9. Learn more about what to do at the Feingold Association of the United States: http://www.feingold.org/research.php   and http://www.feingold.org/newsletters.php. Free email newsletter available at: http://www.feingold.org/ON.html.

10. McCann D, Barrett A, Cooper A et al. Food additives and hyperactive behaviour in 3-year-old and 8/9-year-old children in the community: a randomised, double-blinded, placebo-controlled trial. *Lancet.* 2007 Nov 3;370(9598):1560–7.

Chapter 11: How to Improve a Child's Behavior Without Drugs

1. Dr. Thomas W. Phelan. http://www.thomasphelan.com.

2. Gesch, C.B., S.M. Hammond, S.E. Hampson, et al. "Influence of Supplementary Vitamins, Minerals and Essential Fatty Acids on the Antisocial Behaviour of Young Adult Prisoners. Randomised, Placebo-controlled Trial." *Br J Psychiatry* 181 (July 2002): 22–28.

3. Saul, A.W. "Interview with Paul and Barbara Reed Stitt." *Doctor Yourself Newsletter* 5:1 (December 2004). http://www.doctoryourself.com/news/v5n1.html.

Chapter 12: High-Dose Vitamin C Therapy

1. McCormick, W.J. "The Changing Incidence and Mortality of Infectious Disease in Relation to Changed Trends in Nutrition." *Med Record* (September 1947).

2. McCormick, W.J. "Coronary Thrombosis: A New Concept of Mechanism and Etiology." *Clin Med* 4:7 (July 1957).

3. McCormick, W.J. "Intervertebral-disc Lesions: A New Etiological Concept." *Arch Pediatr* 71:1 (January 1954): 29–32.

4. Rath, M., and L. Pauling. "Solution to the Puzzle of Human Cardiovascular Disease: Its Primary Cause Is Ascorbate Deficiency Leading to the Deposition of Lipoprotein(a) and Fibrinogen/Fibrin in the Vascular Wall." *J Orthomolecular Med* 6 (3rd and 4th Quarters 1991): 125. Rath, M., and L. Pauling. "A Unified Theory of Human Cardiovascular Disease Leading the Way To the Abolition of This Diseases as a Cause for Human Mortality." *J Orthomolecular Med* 7 (1st Quarter 1992): 5.

5. Chen, Q., et al. "Pharmacologic Doses of Ascorbate Act as a Pro-oxidant and Decrease Growth of Aggressive Tumor Xenografts in Mice." *Proc Natl Acad Sci USA* (August 2008).

6. McCormick, W.J. "Cancer: The Preconditioning Factor in Pathogenesis." *Arch Pediatr N Y* 71 (1954): 313.

7. Klenner, F.R. "Observations on the Dose of Administration of Ascorbic Acid When Employed Beyond the Range of a Vitamin in Human Pathology." *J Appl Nutr* 23:3–4 (1971): 61–68. Available online at: http://www.doctoryourself.com/klennerpaper.html.

CHAPTER 275

8. Klenner, F.R. "Response of Peripheral and Central Nerve Pathology to Mega-doses of the Vitamin B-complex and Other Metabolites. Parts 1 and 2." *J Appl Nutr* 25 (1973): 16–40. Available for download at: http://www.townsendletter .com/Klenner/KlennerProtocol_forMS.pdf.

9. Cathcart, R.F. "Vitamin C, Titration to Bowel Tolerance, Anascorbemia, and Acute Induced Scurvy." *Med Hypotheses* 7 (1981): 1359–1376. Available online at: http://www.doctoryourself.com/titration.html. Cathcart, R.F. "Vitamin C in the Treatment of Acquired Immune Deficiency Syndrome (AIDS)." *Med Hypotheses* 14:4 (1984): 423–433. Cathcart, R.F. "Vitamin C, the Nontoxic, Nonrate-limited Antioxidant Free Radical Scavenger." *Med Hypotheses* 18 (1985): 61–77.

10. Riordan, H.D. "The Use of Vitamin C Infusions in Cancer (1975–2002)." *Vitamin C Cancer* (November 2002).

11. Williams, R.J., and G. Deason. "Individuality in Vitamin C Needs." *Proc Natl Acad Sci USA* 57 (1967): 1638–1641. Pauling, L. *How to Live Longer and Feel Better.* Corvallis, OR: Oregon State University Press, 2006. Hoffer, A., and A.W. Saul. *Orthomolecular Medicine for Everyone: Megavitamin Therapeutics for Families and Physicians.* Laguna Beach, CA: Basic Health, 2009.

12. Levy, T.E. *Curing the Incurable: Vitamin C, Infectious Diseases, and Toxins.* Henderson, NV: Livon Books, 2002. Hickey, S., and A.W. Saul. *Vitamin C: The Real Story, The Remarkable and Controversial Healing Factor.* Laguna Beach, CA: Basic Health, 2008.

13. Hickey, S., and A.W. Saul. *Vitamin C: The Real Story, The Remarkable and Controversial Healing Factor.* Laguna Beach, CA: Basic Health, 2008.

14. Hickey, S., and A.W. Saul. *Vitamin C: The Real Story, The Remarkable and Controversial Healing Factor.* Laguna Beach, CA: Basic Health, 2008. Cathcart, R.F. "Vitamin C, Titrating to Bowel Tolerance, Anascorbemia, and Acute Induced Scurvy." *Med Hypotheses* 7 (1981): 1359–1376.

15. Levy, T.E. *Curing the Incurable: Vitamin C, Infectious Diseases, and Toxins.* Henderson, NV: Livon Books, 2002. Hickey, S., and A.W. Saul. *Vitamin C: The Real Story, The Remarkable and Controversial Healing Factor.* Laguna Beach, CA: Basic Health, 2008. Klenner, F.R. (1979) "The Significance of High Daily Intake of Ascorbic Acid in Preventive Medicine." In: Williams, R., and D. Kalita (eds.). *A Physician's Handbook on Orthomolecular Medicine,* 3rd edition. New York: Pergamon, 1977, pp. 51–59.

16. Levy, T.E. *Curing the Incurable: Vitamin C, Infectious Diseases, and Toxins.* Henderson, NV: Livon Books, 2002. Webb, A.L., and E. Villamor. "Update: Effects of Antioxidant and Non-antioxidant Vitamin Supplementation on Immune Function." *Nutr Rev* 65 (2007): 181–217.

17. Wintergerst, E.S., S. Maggini, D.H. Hornig. "Immune-enhancing Role of Vitamin C and Zinc and Effect on Clinical Conditions." *Ann Nutr Metab* 50 (2006): 85–94.

18. Kastenbauer, S., U. Koedel, B.F. Becker, H.W. Pfister. "Oxidative Stress in Bacterial Meningitis in Humans." *Neurology* 58 (2002): 186–191.

19. Murata, A., R. Oyadomari, T. Ohashi, K. Kitagawa. "Mechanism of Inactivation of Bacteriophage Delta A Containing Single-stranded DNA by Ascorbic Acid." *J Nutr Sci Vitaminol (Tokyo)* 21 (1975): 261–269. Harakeh, S., R.J. Jariwalla, L. Pauling. "Suppression of Human Immunodeficiency Virus Replication by Ascorbate in Chronically and Acutely Infected Cells." *Proc Natl Acad Sci USA* 87 (1990): 7245–7249. White, L.A., C.Y. Freeman, B.D. Forrester, W.A. Chappell. "In Vitro Effect of Ascorbic Acid on Infectivity of Herpesviruses and Paramyxoviruses." *J Clin Microbiol* 24 (1986): 527–531.

20. Furuya, A., M. Uozaki, H. Yamasaki, et al. "Antiviral Effects of Ascorbic and Dehydroascorbic Acids in Vitro." *Int J Mol Med* 22 (2008): 541–545.

21. Gerber, W.F. "Effect of Ascorbic Acid, Sodium Salicylate and Caffeine on the Serum Interferon Level in Response to Viral Infection." *Pharmacology* 13 (1975): 228. Karpinska, T., Z. Kawecki, M. Kandefer-Szerszen. "The Influence of Ultraviolet Irradiation, L-Ascorbic Acid and Calcium Chloride on the Induction of Interferon in Human Embryo Fibroblasts." *Arch Immunol Ther Exp (Warsz)* 30 (1982): 33–37.

22. Anderson, R., and O.C. Dittrich. "Effects of Ascorbate on Leucocytes: Part IV. Increased Neutrophil Function and Clinical Improvement After Oral Ascorbate in 2 Patients with Chronic Granulomatous Disease." *S Afr Med J* 56:12 (1979): 476–480.

23. Gonzalez, M.J., J.R. Miranda, H.D. Riordan. "Vitamin C as an Ergogenic Aid." *J Orthomolecular Med* 20 (2005): 100–102.

24. Levy, T.E. *Curing the Incurable: Vitamin C, Infectious Diseases, and Toxins.* Henderson, NV: Livon Books, 2002.

25. Ibid.

26. Kennes, B., I. Dumont, D. Brohee, et al. "Effect of Vitamin C Supplements on Cell-mediated Immunity in Old People." *Gerontology* 29 (1983): 305–310. Siegel, B.V., and J.I. Morton. "Vitamin C and Immunity: Influence of Ascorbate on Prostaglandin E2 Synthesis and Implications for Natural Killer Cell Activity." *Int J Vitam Nutr Res* 54 (1984): 339–342. Jeng, K.C., C.S. Yang, W.Y. Siu, et al. "Supplementation with Vitamins C and E Enhances Cytokine Production by Peripheral Blood Mononuclear Cells in Healthy Adults." *Am J Clin Nutr* 64 (1996): 960–965. Campbell, J.D., M. Cole, B. Bunditrutavorn, A.T. Vella. "Ascorbic Acid is a Potent Inhibitor of Various Forms of T-cell Apoptosis." *Cell Immunol* 194 (1999): 1–5. Schwager, J., and J. Schulze. "Influence of Ascorbic Acid on the Response to Mitogens and Interleukin Production of Porcine Lymphocytes." *Int J Vitam Nutr Res* 67 (1997): 10–16.

27. Banic, S. "Immunostimulation by Vitamin C." *Int J Vitam Nutr Res Suppl* 23 (1982): 49–52. Wu, C.C., T. Dorairajan, T.L. Lin. "Effect of Ascorbic Acid Supplementation on the Immune Response of Chickens Vaccinated and Challenged with Infectious Bursal Disease Virus." *Vet Immunol Immunopathol* 74 (2000): 145–152.

28. Clemetson, C.A.B. "Vaccinations, Inoculations and Ascorbic Acid." *J Orthomolecular Med* 14:3 (Third Quarter 1999).

CHAPTER 277

29. Padayatty, S.J., H. Sun, Y. Wang, et al. "Vitamin C Pharmacokinetics: Implications for Oral and Intravenous Use." *Ann Intern Med* 140:7 (April 2004): 533–537.

30. Klenner, F.R. "The Significance of High Daily Intake of Ascorbic Acid in Preventive Medicine." In: Williams, R., and D. Kalita (eds.). *A Physician's Handbook on Orthomolecular Medicine*, 3rd edition. New York: Pergamon, 1977, pp. 51–59.

31. Pauling, L. *How to Live Longer and Feel Better.* Corvallis, OR: Oregon State University Press, 2006. Linus Pauling's complete vitamin and nutrition bibliography is posted at: http://www.doctoryourself.com/biblio_pauling_ortho.html. The complete text of Irwin Stone's book *The Healing Factor* is posted at: http://vitamincfoundation.org/stone/.

32. "No Deaths from Vitamins, Minerals, Amino Acids, or Herbs." Orthomolecular Medicine News Service (January 19, 2010); http://orthomolecular.org/resources/omns/v06n04.shtml.

33. Levine, M., et al. *JAMA* 281:15 (April 1999): 1419.

34. McCormick, W.J. "Lithogenesis and Hypovitaminosis." *Med Record* 159:7 (July 1946): 410–413.

35. Cheraskin, E., M. Ringsdorf Jr., E. Sisley. *The Vitamin C Connection: Getting Well and Staying Well with Vitamin C.* New York: Harper and Row, 1983. See also: Ringsdorf Jr., W.M., and E. Cheraskin. "Nutritional Aspects of Urolithiasis." *South Med J* 74:1 (January 1981): 41–43, 46.

36. Curhan, G.C., W.C. Willett, F.E. Speizer, M.J. Stampfer. "Megadose Vitamin C Consumption Does Not Cause Kidney Stones. Intake of Vitamins B6 and C and the Risk of Kidney Stones in Women." *J Am Soc Nephrol* 10:4 (April 1999): 840–845.

37. Gerster, H. "No Contribution of Ascorbic Acid to Renal Calcium Oxalate Stones." *Ann Nutr Metab* 41:5 (1997): 269–282. See also: "Vitamin C Does Not Cause Kidney Stones." Orthomolecular Medicine News Service (July 5, 2005); http://orthomolecular.org/resources/omns/v01n07.shtml.

38. See: Gokce, N., J.F. Keaney, Jr., B. Frei, et al. "Long-Term Ascorbic Acid Administration Reverses Endothelial Vasomotor Dysfunction in Patients With Coronary Artery Disease." *Circulation* 99 (1999): 3234–3240; free full-text paper at: http://circ.ahajournals.org/cgi/reprint/99/25/3234. See also: "About 'Objections' to Vitamin C Therapy." Orthomolecular Medicine News Service (October 12, 2010); http://orthomolecular.org/resources/omns/v06n24.shtml. "Vitamin C and Cardiovascular Disease." Orthomolecular Medicine News Service (June 22, 2010); http://orthomolecular.org/ resources/omns/v06n20.shtml. "Vitamin C Saves Lives." Orthomolecular Medicine News Service (April 22, 2005); http://orthomolecular.org/resources/omns/v01n02.shtml.

39. Ivanov, V.O., S.V. Ivanova, A. Niedzwiecki. "Ascorbate Affects Proliferation of Guinea-pig Vascular Smooth Muscle Cells by Direct and Extracellular Matrix-mediated Effects." *J Mol Cell Cardiol* 29:12 (December 1997): 3293–3303. See

also: Ivanov, V.O., et al. "Transforming Growth Factor-beta 1 and Ascorbate Regulate Proliferation of Cultured Smooth Muscle Cells by Independent Mechanisms." *Atherosclerosis* 140:1 (September 1998): 25–34.

Chapter 13: Vitamin D and Other Supplements

1. "Doctors say, Raise the RDAs Now." Orthomolecular Medicine News Service (October 30, 2007); http://orthomolecular.org/resources/omns/v03n10.shtml.

2. "Interview with Michael Holick, M.D." DoctorYourself.com. http://www.doctoryourself.com/holick.html.

3. Ibid.

4. Bacon, C.J., G.D. Gamble, A.M. Horne, et al. "High-dose Oral Vitamin D3 Supplementation in the Elderly." *Osteoporos Int* 20:8 (August 2009): 1407–1415.

5. Rosenberg, H., and A.N. Feldzamen. *The Book of Vitamin Therapy.* New York: Berkley, 1974, p. 98.

6. Bronstein, A.C., D.A. Spyker, L.R. Cantilena Jr., et al. "2008 Annual Report of the American Association of Poison Control Centers' National Poison Data System (NPDS): 26th Annual Report." *Clin Toxicol* 47 (2009): 911–1084. The full text is available for download at: http://www.aapcc.org/dnn/Portals/0/2008annualreport.pdf. Vitamin statistics are found in Table 22B, pp. 1052–1053; minerals, herbs, amino acids, and other supplements are in the same table, pp. 1047–1048.

7. Leape, L. "Error in Medicine." *JAMA* 272:23 (1994): 1851. Also: Leape, L.L. "Institute of Medicine Medical Error Figures are Not Exaggerated." *JAMA* 284:1 (July 2000): 95–97.

INDEX

ABOUT THE AUTHORS

Ralph Campbell, M.D., is a life-long advocate of nutritional medicine. He grew up in Long Beach, California, received his medical degree from Yale University Medical School in 1954, and completed his residency in pediatrics at Los Angeles Children's Hospital. He maintained a large pediatric practice in Southern California for thirteen years, then moved to Polson, Montana, in 1970. Dr. Campbell conducted well-child clinics for the Salish Kootenai Reservation, established the Lake County Health Department, had a private pediatric practice, and served as a county jail doctor. His wide experience continues to inform and invigorate his steady commitment to nutritionally oriented medicine, which has endured through numerous cultural changes in the medical community.

Andrew W. Saul, Ph.D., has taught nutrition, health science, and cell biology at the college level. He is the author of *Doctor Yourself* and *Fire Your Doctor!* (both from Basic Health Publications). With Dr. Abram Hoffer, he co-wrote *Orthomolecular Medicine for Everyone* and *The Vitamin Cure for Alcoholism.* He is also co-author of three other books: *Vitamin C: The Real Story, I Have Cancer: What Should I Do?,* and *Hospitals and Health* (all available from Basic Health). Dr. Saul is on the editorial board of the *Journal of Orthomolecular Medicine* and is featured in the documentary film *Food Matters.* He has published over 100 reviews and editorials in peer-reviewed publications. His internationally famous, non-commercial, natural healing website is www.DoctorYourself.com.

CPSIA information can be obtained
at www.ICGtesting.com
Printed in the USA
LVOW13*2249220418
574485LV00011B/49/P